SOARING to SUCCESS

Taking Crew Resource Management from
the Cockpit to the Nursing Unit

Gary L. Sculli, RN, MSN, ATP
David M. Sine, MA, CSP, ARM, CPHRM

HCPro

Gary L. Sculli, RN, MSN, ATP, Author
David M. Sine, MA, CSP, ARM, CPHRM, Author
Rebecca Hendren, Senior Managing Editor
Mike Briddon, Executive Editor
Emily Sheahan, Group Publisher

Mike Mirabello, Senior Graphic Artist
Matt Sharpe, Production Supervisor
Shane Katz, Art Director
Jean St. Pierre, Senior Director of Operations

Advice given is general. Readers should consult professional counsel for specific legal, ethical, or clinical questions. Arrangements can be made for quantity discounts. For more information, contact:

HCPro, Inc.
75 Sylvan Street, Suite A-101
Danvers, MA 01923
Telephone: 800/650-6787 or 781/639-1872
Fax: 781/639-7857
E-mail: *customerservice@hcpro.com*

Visit HCPro online at: *www.hcpro.com* and *www.hcmarketplace.com*

Rev. 04/2013
52899

Contents

About the Authors

Gary L. Sculli, RN, MSN, ATP

Gary L. Sculli, RN, MSN, ATP, brings a unique and diverse perspective to patient safety with his background as both a clinician and an airline pilot. He has been a registered nurse since 1986 and has practiced in multiple clinical specialties including medicine, general surgery, ENT oncology, orthopedic surgery, neurology, and neurosurgery. He has experience as a nurse educator, nurse manager, and completed a tour of duty as an officer in the United States Air Force Nurse Corps, Lackland Air Force Base, TX.

Sculli is also a former airline pilot with experience flying turboprop and jet aircraft at the regional and major/global airline level. His flying background includes experience as a captain, first officer, and aircrew instructor, and FAA certified line check airman. He has conducted airline training in state-of-the-art aircraft simulators and has developed and taught airline crew resource management (CRM) programs.

Sculli currently works in patient safety at a national level. He is an accomplished presenter and patient safety consultant. He has extensive experience developing and delivering clinical programs that apply CRM and human factors concepts directly to frontline nursing practice and interdisciplinary healthcare teams.

He holds an airline transport pilot certificate with three type ratings. He received a BSN from Thomas Jefferson University in Philadelphia and an MSN from The University of Memphis.

David M. Sine, MA, CSP, ARM, CPHRM

David M. Sine, MA, CSP, ARM, CPHRM, has more than 30 years of healthcare safety and risk management experience in private and public sector health systems. He currently serves as a member of Joint Commission's Committee on Healthcare Safety, and acts as a risk management and patient safety advisor to the National Association of Psychiatric Health Systems.

Sine was formerly a senior staff engineer for The Joint Commission, a senior consultant for the American Hospital Association, and a vice chair of the board of Brackenridge Hospital in Austin, TX. He was the inaugural contributing editor for *Briefings on Hospital Safety*, published by HCPro, Inc., and *Quality Improvement Techniques for Hospital Safety*, and is the coauthor of the *Design Guide for Behavioral Health Facilities*, published by the National Association of Psychiatric Health Systems.

He is a past chair of the American Society for Healthcare Risk Management ethics committee (2009), and has been the Spencer Educational Foundation risk manager in residence. He has published numerous articles and is a frequent speaker at national and regional educational programs.

His research interest is the intersection of risk management, patient safety, and ethics. He holds a degree from the School of the Art Institute of Chicago (SAIC) in design and from Loyola University in bioethics and health policy. He divides his time between Ann Arbor, MI, and Austin, TX.

How to Read
This Book

This book is designed to give you an overview of nursing culture and an explanation of crew resource management and airline safety practices in the first two chapters. Chapters 3 and onward provide practical discussion of various principles that you can use to improve communication, leadership, and safety practices on patient care units.

It is entirely acceptable to read the book in page order, but it is also acceptable to skip ahead to a specific chapter if you have a particular interest in its content and do not want to wait. The chapters are designed to flow consecutively, but they are also self-contained modules that stand alone nicely.

You will notice numbered sidebars written by the book's coauthor, David Sine, arising from the main body of text within the chapters. Much of the book is written in narrative form. The narrative content is based on my experience and current literature. To a much larger degree, the sidebars provide an academic and literature/research base contribution that strengthens the manuscript.

However you choose to proceed, we hope you will use the book as a reference long into the future.

Gary L. Sculli, RN, MSN, ATP

Continuing Education Credits Available

Continuing education credits are available for this book for two years from date of purchase.

For more information about credits available, and to take the continuing education exam, please see the Nursing Education Instructional Guide found with the downloadable resources at *www.hcpro.com/downloads/8993.*

Acknowledgments

Thank you to Anita Garrison, RN, MSN, CPHQ, a true mentor who recognized the importance of this work long before I did. I am <u>forever</u> grateful. Also to Cheryl Rice, RN, BSN, for your innovative mind and thoughtful guidance.

Thank you Dr. Jim Bagian for your support of CRM in nursing practice. Many thanks to Dr. Douglas E. Paull for your consultation and expertise.

Thanks to David Sine for your partnership.

Most of all, thank you Lauren, Peter, and Elizabeth for your love and patience.

Gary L. Sculli, RN, MSN, ATP

Many colleagues, friends, reviewers, faculty, and clients have influenced this work. I cannot name them all, but for providing good counsel, reading countless drafts, and helping to keep me on track, I am especially grateful to Dr.'s Mike Cornett and Norvell Northcutt at Texas State and The University of Texas respectively, Dr. Kathleen McCann at NAPHS, Jim Hunt, Bob Keyburn, John McKillop, Carrie Baker, a gaggle of Grosenheiders, Kara Clark at ASHRM, Ed and Kate West at the University of Michigan, and last, but not least, The Bev.

David M. Sine, MA, CSP, ARM, CPHRM

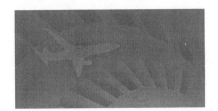

Foreword

For more than a decade, patient safety has glowed brightly on the radar screen of not only health professionals but also on the radar screen of the media and patients. There has been no shortage of catastrophic events that have appeared on the front page of newspapers or been the subject of media coverage documenting tragedies that have affected patients in the course of their healthcare. Examination of the root causes and contributing factors that led up to these terrible events have consistently identified communication as the most common underlying causative factor. The critical role of communication is common to most human activities and is not unique to healthcare. When communication problems arise in the majority of human activities, the result is not the death of the participants. There are, however, some industrial, commercial, and professional activities in which the penalty for communication failures is death or major injury. Aviation and healthcare are two such endeavors in which the penalty for less than clear and effective communication can be catastrophic.

Authors Gary Sculli and David Sine have taken advantage of the opportunity to contrast the aviation industry and how it effectively dealt with communication challenges through the use of crew resource management-based techniques, with the general lack of coherent practices to deal with similar communication problems in healthcare. This book illustrates how principles and lessons learned in the aviation environment such as structured communication, checklists, teamwork, task sharing, situation awareness, and elements of human factors can be applied to the challenges presented in healthcare. The authors have clearly understood that there is no magic bullet to deal with the challenges in today's high-risk and technologically complex healthcare environment and have taken a systems-based approach to provide a useful multipronged methodology. This variety of techniques equips the reader with a formidable armamentarium to deal effectively with communication challenges on the nursing unit and may assist in providing higher quality and safer patient care than in the past.

Until recently, healthcare did not fully recognize the profound effect flawed communication could have on patient care and, even more importantly, did not routinely have access to the tools to assist in dealing with these issues. *Soaring to Success*, through the use of engaging personal examples from the authors' own unique experiences in aviation and healthcare and well researched references, gives us such a tool.

James P. Bagian, MD, PE
Director, Center for Health Engineering and Patient Safety
Chief Patient Safety and Systems Innovation Officer
University of Michigan
Founding Director, VA National Center for Patient Safety

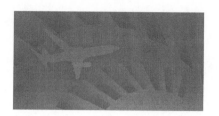

Preface

September 11, 2001, changed many lives. It irrevocably changed mine. I will never, as long as I live, stop reflecting on what happened to the victims that day and what they endured, especially those who experienced unimaginable terror on those airplanes. I admit, as the years slip by, my pensive moments about this apocalyptic event come less often; but as is the case with so many of us, I will never forget what happened, and I doubt that I will ever get to the point that it does not affect me viscerally.

On September 10, 2001, I flew as first officer on a Northwest Airlines DC-9 from Minneapolis-St. Paul to Memphis, TN. We arrived around 1200 central time after an early start in Minot, ND. How could I possibly know that this would be the last landing for me where life as an airline pilot seemed so full of promise? It seems tragically ironic that on the day prior, while in my hotel room, I watched the Secretary of Defense Donald Rumsfeld appear on one of the Sunday news shows talk about Israel and terrorism. He explained that the Israelis had a much greater problem in dealing with terrorism than we did here in the United States, because unlike us, it surrounded them. The fact that it occurred in their country, on their soil, mandated that they deal harshly with acts of terror and violence. As Mr. Rumsfeld said this, it was implied, even taken for granted, that we were insulated from such things here in the United States. Little did we know what was headed our way.

In the days following the attacks of 9/11, it became apparent that I was going to be laid off from the airline. I was at the bottom of the seniority list, and in the airline world, seniority is job protection. As time went on, I saw that the layoff was going to be protracted, so I prepared to re-enter nursing, a profession I had practiced for nine years before transitioning to the airlines. Although I had practiced in multiple clinical specialties on all shifts—both as a military officer and civilian employee—I did not anticipate the experience that awaited me.

My first position upon my return to nursing was as a nurse educator with a local healthcare system. Half of my time was spent teaching new hire orientation, which I enjoyed thoroughly, and the other half as a unit-based educator on an oncology unit. It was here that I began to realize my view of nursing as a profession had changed and that I now approached it from a completely different perspective. I was looking at nursing through a different prism. When I later moved into nursing leadership as a frontline nurse manager, this realization was reinforced.

This book is about that very realization: transitioning from an industry that consistently functions and perpetuates a culture of safety, back into nursing, a noble profession that articulates desired patient outcomes quite well, but often fails to provide its personnel with the tools, resources, and environmental conditions for such outcomes to take place.

I firmly believe that clinical nursing, especially in the multibed medical-surgical specialty, will benefit enormously from the application of some of the most basic tenets of crew resource management (CRM), a program that has transformed the airline industry and changed the manner in which flight crews interact to ensure passenger safety. CRM can transform nursing practice at the front line as well. I have seen this firsthand. It facilitates environmental changes, clinical processes, staff attitudes, and behaviors that hold true to the edict "first do no harm."

In addition, the airline industry has other safeguards and supplemental practices that ensure operational safety, which can be combined with CRM and exported to nursing practice.

In a sense, this book is a second chance. During my first tenure in nursing, I felt uneasy and frankly dissatisfied with many of the cultural norms and processes in place. Not only did the culture create vulnerabilities for patient safety, it also induced profound stress and dissatisfaction for the many professional nurses who tirelessly dedicated themselves to caring for the sick. These realizations were clear to me; yet I wasn't sure how to fix these problems. I admit I stepped back and left the profession, as so many nurses do. Call it a divine plan or call it fate, but I had a chance to come back to the profession with knowledge I did not have before, a chance to offer solutions that can make a difference for nurses and patients.

The book is written by a nurse who happens to be a former airline pilot, not the other way around. This is an important point. This book's premise is not that aviation is the savior that has finally arrived to fix the ills within professional nursing. On the contrary; a fundamental paradigm here is that nurses are not pilots and patients are not airplanes. CRM concepts must first be modified to fit the unique environment and culture in which nurses practice, then applied to the clinical area. The differences between the unpredictable world of patient care and the often controlled and knowable responses of aircraft must be taken into account. Simply dropping in aviation tools and practices on the nursing unit without adaptation will not work. That said, there is much to learn from the airlines, a decidedly reliable, safety-sensitive industry that enjoys a high degree of operational safety.

I am a nurse. I have lived in the culture and intimately understand the pressures and forces that affect a nurse's ability to keep his or her patients safe. I am also a pilot. I have lived in the culture and understand the dynamic environment that defines the airline cockpit. Please join me as we go from the cockpit to the nursing unit, a journey that ultimately benefits our patients.

Gary L. Sculli, RN, MSN, ATP

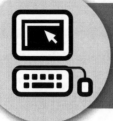

DOWNLOAD YOUR MATERIALS NOW

All the tools and templates in the book are online so you can adapt and use them at your facility. The files are available as Word documents so they may be easily customized and are organized by figure number in the book. You can find the tools online at the website listed below.

www.hcpro.com/downloads/8993

Thank you for purchasing this product!

HCPro

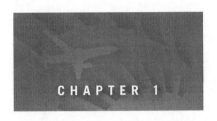

Nursing and Aviation: A Culture Comparison

The purpose of this chapter is to provide an overview of two professional cultures: aviation and nursing. It is important to remember that this overview is general in nature and largely based on my experience and perspective as I moved from the cockpit to the nursing unit. More detailed discussions of the concepts mentioned here occur in later chapters and will be referenced accordingly.

The airline culture is not perfect. Nothing involving human endeavor ever will be. It is, however, what I consider a true culture of safety. When I left the cockpit in 2002 and returned to nursing, I quickly reacclimated to the language and flow of the profession. But, this time something was clearly different, and I knew it right away. My cultural paradigm had completely changed. My expectations for nursing regarding levels of standardization, training, task load management, and communication styles were not the same as before. As I compared my experiences in the cockpit and my indoctrination into the airline culture to what I was currently encountering as a nurse,

I soon realized that I was in a state of culture shock, plain and simple. Reality was not matching my expectations. ◆

I have always known that nurses are dedicated professionals who strive for excellence, yet now I was perplexed, even alarmed, at how many of us—at all levels of practice (including nurse leaders)—accepted vast shortcomings in the culture with regard to patient safety.

◆ Sidebar 1.1
Characteristics of professions

Pilots and nurses share the basic characteristics of all professions. Namely, the expertise of the professional member has been validated by the community of his or her peers, the necessary knowledge and competence to be a member rests on scientific grounds, and the profession's members are oriented by a shared set of normative values.[1] The method of gaining entry to the ranks of pilots and nurses is also similar to that of other professions in that the unique knowledge and skills demanded by both professions are sufficiently esoteric that education and experience can only be gained under the direction of someone who is already an expert.[2]

There seemed to be a palpable sense of resignation when discussions of these shortcomings emerged. For example, I would often hear stories or witness firsthand situations in which physicians purposely intimidated nurses during the course of communicating clinical information. Sometimes there would be yelling, berating in front of patients and families, pointing of fingers, tossing of objects, sarcastic responses to questions, hanging up the phone, and … well, the list goes on.

I knew this type of behavior existed on nursing units. I experienced it myself while practicing years earlier, but now it seemed unimaginable to me and I could not accept it. I would fervently discuss, with anyone who would listen, the simple fact that these communication patterns drastically undermine patient safety and should not be tolerated.[3] I would go on to describe how in the cockpit such behavior would be considered deviant, not common place, and was trained out of the culture long ago. Although many nurses agreed, all too often they would slowly shake their heads back and forth as if to say, "I hear you and I concur, but that's just the way it is."

How could this be? How can a culture with so much at stake function successfully when people—who are supposed to be on the same team, working toward the same goals—cannot talk to each other? How can a culture proclaim that it is safe when some professional groups within it are afraid to speak up if they see a problem or have a question? Communication was not the only cultural challenge that struck me this way. There were many others, and collectively they are deeply problematic for nurses as they care for their patients on nursing units.

This is in no way an indictment of nurses or nursing. On the contrary, it is simply an acknowledgment of the disconnect I experienced after honestly assessing the systems and culture that define professional nursing when compared to a high-reliability industry like aviation—and that is the key here. Nurses are perceptive and smart. I was not pointing out anything they had not already endured or seen. The difference, however, was that I had spent years in a safety-sensitive industry and seen it done in a different way, with excellent results. There are many similarities among nurses and pilots. They are both responsible for the safety of other human beings, and they operate in situations where mistakes can mean the difference between successful outcomes or loss of life. Culturally, however, there are significant differences. ◆

In my mind I envisioned a blank page with a thick black line down the center. On one

> ◆ Sidebar 1.2
> ## Preserving a group's culture
>
> Of the numerous (and arguably equally valid) operating theories and definitions of culture, nearly all share one common aspect: the idea that certain things in social groups are shared or held in common.[4] Behaviors by group members reinforce these values and members tend to behave in ways that teach these practices to new members, rewarding those who fit in and sanctioning those who do not. In this manner, the group behavior persists and the values are preserved over time even when group membership changes.[5]
>
> For new group members, the central-most values of an organization are at first as opaque and mysterious as they are to any outsider. For the newcomer, the threat of punishment for irregular behavior is possibly a more significant motivator than any vague perception of a potential reward that awaits attainment of "insider" status granted though a shared taxonomy and knowledge of the organization's symbols, rituals, and stories.[6]

side was the airline culture, and on the other side nursing. As I filled in the description of the cultures on each side of that line, stark contrasts emerged. Let us compare the two cultures.

Aviation Side of the Line

Team

At the airlines, there is a heavy emphasis on team training and team-building behaviors in the cockpit and beyond. This is the very essence of crew resource management (CRM), a program that has at its core the essential skills required to promote teamwork and effective communication (see Chapter 2 for a detailed explanation of CRM).

Teamwork and team-oriented behaviors are not only discussed in the classroom, they are reinforced and applied during flight simulation training sessions. Each member of the crew has specific responsibilities for keeping the team intact and functioning so that important flight information is communicated in a timely and effective manner. It is understood that while leaders ultimately make operational decisions, all members of the team must participate and play an active role in the decision-making process. This is not only encouraged, it is expected. As leaders, airline captains fully assume the fundamental responsibility of building and maintaining the team. In large part, their effectiveness as leaders determines the effectiveness of the crew as a whole. To that end, captains learn and implement specific behaviors to ensure their team is engaged and speaking up when necessary (see Chapter 4 for a detailed discussion of leadership and team-building behaviors).

CRM training also emphasizes the other side of the team equation, focusing on the crucial roles and responsibilities of those who support the captain. Subordinate crew members learn to use tools that allow them to communicate information effectively and assert their concerns to gain clear resolution when safety is in question. In the cockpit, followers are equally responsible for team outcomes (see Chapter 6 for a complete discussion of effective followership).

From the date of hire at an airline and through initial training, new pilot hires are paired and train together as a crew. As they move through the various phases of simulator training, the crew understands that while each member is being evaluated individually, their ability to successfully complete training depends in large part on how well they work together as a team. Pilots carry this with them beyond the training environment. They know full well that a strong sense of team, coupled with open communication, is their most effective tool in managing error and avoiding mishaps. As we discuss in Chapter 3, the definition of the airline team is not confined to the cockpit, but includes many other players such as flight attendants and maintenance personnel. The key point is that the team umbrella is large enough to ensure that the observations and contributions of those outside the cockpit are not ignored.

Human factors

Another important focal point in the airline culture is an awareness of human factors and the limitations of human performance (also included in CRM training). ◆

This is generally discussed within the context of situational awareness (see Chapter 7 for a full discussion of situational awareness). Specifically, pilots are taught to be acutely aware of fatigue and its effect on

> ◆ Sidebar 1.3
>
> ### A whole-systems approach to human factors
>
> Human factors have come to mean almost exclusively the human machine interface. However, in this book, the term "human factors" refers to the processes and factors that influence the behavior of people.[7] The full scope of human factors research may involve the human-to-human or human-to-environment interface in any work environment and include the disciplines of cognitive and perceptual psychology, engineering, architecture, industrial design, statistics, operations research, and anthropometry. No matter what interface is of interest, the goal of human factors inquiry is to understand and minimize incompatibility between people and the things we create and use.[8, 9]

crew performance and decision making. There is regulatory protection in place, which mandates how long a pilot can be at the controls in a single day, how long a pilot can be available and on duty, and how much rest must occur between duty periods. Although

Soaring to Success

these protections are not foolproof, these Federal Aviation Administration–mandated protections do exist and they are strictly followed. Pilots at most airlines have the option to "call in" fatigued without penalty if they feel that they cannot fly safely. While this option should be used judiciously, it is an available safeguard and can identify systems issues that may create patterns of fatigue among flight crews. ◆

◆ Sidebar 1.4

Patient safety and fatigue

Patient safety studies have shown that hospital nurses have significantly decreased levels of alertness and an increased likelihood for errors and close calls when working extended shifts.[10, 11] The detrimental effects of fatigue also include negative effects on personal health, job performance, and professionalism. Long and often unpredictable hours to cover staffing vacancies, minimal recuperation time, and often unrealistic workloads appear to be a contributing factor in nurse absenteeism and job dissatisfaction.[12] One study found that job dissatisfaction among hospital nurses was four times greater than the average for all workers in the United States.[13]

Incorporated into general operating manuals are information on restrictions surrounding the use of alcohol, strategies to optimize the use of caffeine, and how the ingestion of these substances can affect the ability to obtain restful sleep. The effect of life stressors on performance is openly discussed in the culture. Pilots are encouraged to monitor themselves and each other for the negative effects caused by stress. It is not uncommon for one pilot to ask another who is struggling with a divorce or death of a loved one, "Are you OK to fly today?" The key point is that there is a heightened awareness and active monitoring in the culture for the deleterious effects of stress on performance and operational safety. If it is best for a crew member to be temporarily relieved of flight duties, then that action is within the realm of possibility.

Pilots internalize paradigms and learn procedures that facilitate the safe use of technology as their cockpits become increasingly automated. In addition, there is an unequivocal recognition of the negative effects of distractions on cognitive processes. In the airline cockpit there are rules and procedures that serve to reduce distractions and the effects of extraneous interruptions during critical flight regimes (see Chapter 7 for a complete discussion of the "sterile cockpit" rule). Critical flight regimes are those phases of flight that are task loaded, where vigilance and attention to detail are required to ensure safety. An example of such a regime is when an aircraft is taxiing. While operating on the ground, pilots must maintain awareness of their position relative to other aircraft and active runways, listen and respond to instructions from air traffic control, and complete checklists to ready the aircraft for takeoff. Pilots know well the consequences of losing focus during such times and are expected to remain disciplined and focused throughout.

Human factor awareness is something that emerges at the earliest moments of a pilot's training. For example, when fledgling aviators are first learning to fly an aircraft without visual reference to the natural horizon (called flying by the instruments or flying in instrument meteorological conditions), they must be disciplined enough to ignore the feelings and sensations that their bodies give them and force themselves to rely only on the instruments in front of them. In other words, maintaining aircraft control without the ability to see outside the cockpit requires that pilots respond to what they see inside, not what they feel. Many times the conflicting information between the inner ear and optic nerve can cause overwhelming disorientation. If not managed appropriately, pilots may actually apply pressure on the controls incorrectly without realizing it, placing the aircraft in a dangerous descending spiral. Recall the well-publicized accident of John F. Kennedy Jr., an inexperienced pilot who lost control of his aircraft and plummeted into Nantucket Sound in low visibility. This point underscores the awareness that pilots must possess, almost from the beginning, about the dangers of mismanaging human limitations.

Standardization

Standardization is a staple in the airline industry. There are countless acronyms in the airline vernacular that include the letter "S," which represent the word "standard." Standardized procedures, maneuvers, and actions are ingrained in the culture. In fact, as a pilot, it is the most egregious insult if someone were to describe you professionally as "nonstandard."

Chapter 1

If I were to ask you what is good about standardization, or what does standardization achieve for us as professionals, what would you say? Clearly one answer is that standardization essentially tells us what to do. It ensures that everyone is completing a task or procedure in the same manner. It puts everyone on the same page, reduces variability, and is a critical element in the airline culture. For example, a pilot might fly with 15 different people in a given month. Being standardized means that any two pilots can work together seamlessly in the cockpit and know exactly what to expect from each other regardless of who they are, what their personality types are, or what side of the bed they got up on that morning. It is understood that checklists will be read and responded to in the same way, the aircraft will be configured for takeoff and landing in the same way, and crew callouts and briefings will occur at the same time every time. Who makes up the crew does not affect standard operating procedures. There can be variations in pilot technique and personalities, for sure, but operations are spelled out, everyone is on the same page, and compliance with SOPs is a way of life.

Another important gain from standardization is the fact that it allows us to readily predict behavior. This means that if a crew member does not say or do what he or she is supposed to, when he or she is supposed to, it needs to be investigated immediately. Perhaps this individual is incapacitated, perhaps ill, or maybe fatigued and experiencing low situational awareness. In the cockpit, when someone fails to carry out routine actions as expected, it gets the team's attention.

Some might say that standardization is a bad thing, that it stifles the ability to provide care in a manner that considers each patient as an individual, or that what is good for one is not good for all. I appreciate this concern and would respond this way. First, standards are evidence-based, not arbitrary; it is not wise to practice outside guidelines and protocols derived from data that are results driven. Second, standardization does not preclude considering each patient's individual differences in the implementation of care. For example, a standard may mandate that a nurse conduct preoperative teaching, but how the information is delivered depends solely on the patient's individual method of learning. The standard, preoperative teaching is clearly good for all; the method of delivery is not and therefore is expected to be individualized. Last, standardization also allows for variations in clinician technique when delivering care. Think about the many variations in technique for giving an injection or starting an IV; however, with all of these variations, aseptic standards are still met.

Recurrent training and performance checking through simulation

When pilots are first hired, they go through initial training, part of which is called "indoctrination." Here is where pilots learn the general operating rules and guidelines of the airline. What to do in the case of hijacking, minimum distances to stay clear of thunderstorms, how to handle a sick passenger or bomb threat, proper dress codes, and how much crew rest is required before attempting to fly. Another segment of the initial training is where the pilot learns the systems and cockpit procedures for the particular airplane they are going to fly. This usually includes a combination of classroom and procedure training, which uses static and full motion simulation. The simulator is an exact replica of the cockpit and provides a level of reality that is nothing short of stunning. When pilots emerge from this training, they are ready to go to the line and fly the aircraft with passengers on board. This is where additional training, called initial operating experience (IOE), takes place under the watchful eye of a check airman (just like a preceptor in nursing). When IOE is complete, pilots are released from training and become available to crew scheduling for flying assignments. The entire process takes approximately six weeks.

In the training described, there are points to evaluate a pilot's knowledge and performance. Knowledge testing takes the form of computerized testing and/or oral evaluations. Performance testing takes the form of what is called a check ride. Here, pilots fly the simulator and must demonstrate proficiency and execution of specified aircraft maneuvers within certain tolerances. They also must demonstrate the appropriate management of aircraft emergencies such as an engine failure or rapid depressurization at altitude. The crew is also evaluated on their performance as a team, as they work together to problem solve abnormalities. The check ride is about performance under observation and pilots understand this. Most learn early on in their careers to find ways to manage the natural anxiety that accompanies such an event.

Soaring to Success

As time goes by, pilots become lulled by the normalcy of operations. Aircraft systems and procedures begin to get a bit hazy and difficult to recall. For this reason, the airline industry practices recurrent training and performance checking. This means at specified intervals (every 12 months at a minimum) pilots go back to the classroom to revisit the salient policies and procedures of the airline. They may review important safety topics and lessons learned from industry accidents or mishaps. They review aircraft systems and operating limitations, along with any significant changes to airline procedures. They also complete a recurrent check ride in the simulator as previously described. Recurrent training and performance checking is one method the airline culture uses to manage the natural tendency for human beings to become complacent over time. Pilots emerge from recurrent training with revitalized knowledge and confidence, which creates margins of safety in the operational environment. (For a complete description of recurrent training and performance checking and how it can be applied to nursing practice, see Chapter 9.)

Checklists

Pilots live and die by checklists—literally. Aviation history has its share of mishaps that can be traced back to poor or absent checklist utilization. This is the rare exception, not the rule. I mentioned earlier that standardization is a staple in the airline industry; the same can be said for checklists. Pilots discipline themselves to adhere to checklists consistently and without question. This does not imply that checklists are used without judgment, but it does mean they are consulted at specific points during all phases of flight to support memory and situational awareness.[14] It is not unreasonable to say that checklists are the backbone of the airline safety culture.

Checklists are used differently depending on the situation. For example, the manner in which a pilot uses a checklist in an emergency varies significantly from how it will be used for routine scenarios. In fact, the checklists themselves look different in terms of presentation and structure. Differences in checklist philosophy and presentation ensure ease of use and optimal support of human memory. If you are a nurse who has practiced on the unit, think back to a time that you used a checklist in practice. Was it easy to use? Did it make sense?

Did it make your job easier or create more work for you? As discussion about the use of checklists to support patient safety heats up, nurses will experience increasing pressure to use checklists in practice, which is a good thing. However, it is imperative that nurses develop checklists using the appropriate philosophy, matching the checklist's format to the task at hand. An extensive discussion about creating checklists to best support nursing practice can be found in Chapter 8.

This concludes the overview of the aviation culture, and it's time to move on to nursing. Before we do, I feel the need to quote that famous robot from the TV show *Lost in Space*: "Warning Warning, Danger Danger!" There may some unpleasant reading ahead. As I stated earlier, the aim of this chapter is to provide a quick culture comparison based on my vantage point moving from the flight deck to the nursing unit. It is important to keep that in mind, as well as the fact that while we may identify cultural deficiencies, the book is not about decrying problems, but using CRM to solve them. Now that I have covered aviation, let us look at the nursing side of that big black line dividing the cultural page that I envisioned earlier.

Nursing Side of the Line

Hierarchy

Right away, it was apparent to me when I returned to nursing that there are cultural roadblocks to effective communication. Most salient is the hierarchical nature of relationships between members of the patient care team on the nursing unit. Although nurses have information transfer failures within their own team structure, the most clear and present danger to patients can be found in the intense authority gradients existing within the nurse-physician dyad. History demonstrates that, in general, healthcare relationships have been characterized not by open communication and team orientation, but by an emphasis on centralized power in decision making.[15] For nurses, this is all too apparent as they often experience adversarial responses, poor behavior, and unpredictable reactions from medical decision makers while attempting to manage patient problems.

Missed meals

In a way, it seems paradoxical that nurses who spend incredible amounts of time in school learning about the physiology of the human body can live in a culture that quietly avoids serious discussions regarding how human limitations affect clinical performance. Let's start with the two most overused letters in the nursing profession today. They are "N" and "L." Put together they read "NL" which stands for "No Lunch." Nurses often complain that they cannot get lunch because they are so busy. Many times this is absolutely true and regrettable. The culture has responded to this problem by offering compensation when meals are missed. Rather than fix the core issue, we allow nursing staff to write "NL" in a pay exception log; nurses may not eat, but they will get paid. For some nurses this insidiously becomes a part of their financial planning as they realize the boost that these two initials can give their paycheck. The human body needs fuel to maintain acceptable blood glucose levels and to nourish organs and tissues properly, most importantly the brain. Yet in professional nursing today, we expect practitioners to make accurate clinical decisions under great pressures, while at the same time going long hours without a proper meal, enjoyed without interruption.

Fatigue

The research on the negative effects of fatigue on motor and cognitive performance is well documented. As discussed, there is regulatory protection in aviation that sets a standard for pilot duty time and rest requirements. In nursing, such protections are not uniformly present, leaving fatigue and rest guidelines up to individual healthcare organizations. These guidelines can be liberal and are often pushed to the limit or creatively ignored to relieve staffing pressures.

Nursing shift patterns tell the story with multiple 12-hour shifts scheduled in a row. The problem here is that multiple 12-hour shifts can lead to chronic fatigue and sleep debt if restful sleep is not obtained between duty periods. During a day in which nurses complete 12-hour shifts, they may actually be awake for as much as 17 hours, assuming they gets up at 5 a.m. and go to bed by 10 p.m. Even in the best scenario in which restful sleep is obtained for the seven full hours remaining before it is time to get up and do it all over again, this routine can be cumulatively exhausting. It is difficult to believe that at 5 p.m. on the third 12-hour day shift in a row, nurses can safely handle the enormous workload and cognitive challenges existing on today's multibed medical surgical units.

Work factors arguing against 12-hour shifts include:

- Heavy physical work

- Demanding, repetitive mental work

- Safety-sensitive work

- Work requiring vigilance[16]

If this is not the quintessential description of nursing, then I don't know what is. If you understand the nursing culture, you know that 12-hour shifts are embraced by many within it. Twelve-hour shifts provide the opportunity to achieve concentrated work schedules and additional time off within the work week. For a workforce that consists of a large proportion of working mothers and many single working mothers bearing the dual responsibility of breadwinner and parent, this scheduling option can be attractive. When you add to this the existence of double shifts (16 hrs), which sometimes occur back to back, double backs (working until 11 p.m. and returning at 6:45 a.m. the next day), excessive amounts of available overtime, coupled with nurse managers desperate to fill staffing holes day to day, the conditions for the perfect storm to create a fatigued workforce are in place.

Task load

Pilots must multitask. There can be times in the cockpit when things get dicey and task load gets to a saturation point. Undoubtedly, pilots in this situation will miss something or not respond appropriately as the amount of stimuli exceeds the brain's capacity to process. It is, of course, advantageous to have another crew member backing you up so that safety critical items are not overlooked. In medical surgical nursing, task saturation occurs all too frequently, which is a great source of error and frustration. ◆ For example, typical medical surgical nurses may have the following occur on the average day within a 30–60 minute period:

- A physician at the nurse's station wants to talk about a patient's vital signs

- A patient requests IV pain medication

- They begin administering routine morning medications to all seven of their patients

- A patient is awaiting discharge teaching

- A new admission has just arrived on the floor and needs to be clinically assessed and processed

- An IV infusion pump alarm is sounding

- A patient calls to complain that his or her IV is leaking at the insertion site

- A patient needs to be sent to surgery

> ◆ Sidebar 1.5
> ## The myth of multitasking
>
> The shorthand used for the human attempt to simultaneously do as many things as possible, as quickly as possible, preferably marshaling the power of as many technologies as possible, is multitasking.[17] Although we may consider ourselves experts in crowding, pressing, packing, and overlapping distinct activities into all-too-finite moments, according to researcher James Poldrack, "We're really built to focus. And when we sort of force ourselves to multitask, we're driving ourselves to perhaps be less efficient in the long run even though it sometimes feels like we're being more efficient".[18, 19] In addition, we can easily become so preoccupied with one task that monitoring of all other tasks is stopped. Even if monitoring does not drop out completely, the quality of monitoring suffers. Although the study of the cognitive processes involved when juggling several tasks concurrently is just beginning, it is known that multitasking is error prone.[20]

- The blood bank calls and says that the first unit of Packed Red Blood Cells (PRBC) to be transfused for a patient is ready for pickup

- The case manager hands them a nursing home transfer form and wants them to fill in the patient's medications and latest vital signs

Clearly, this is a lot to manage in such a short time. I can see many medical surgical nurses reading this and nodding their heads up and down saying, "Yep, that sounds like a routine day for me." The existing professional culture allows the placement of nurses in situations in which the requirement to multitask reaches unmanageable levels, and at the same time demands precision and success. How can we realistically talk about patient safety when task saturation is the order of the day? Unlike pilots in the cockpit, when nurses endure task saturation, there is often no one to back them up to make sure critical things are not overlooked.

Nonnursing functions

Put simply, nurses are often expected to complete nonclinical, nonnursing functions. Let me say it this way: When I was flying in an airliner, never did anyone say to me, "Look guys, today we are short a flight attendant. What I need you to do is when you level off at 35,000 feet, unbuckle you safety harness, walk to the back, and help serve peanuts and ginger ale." It is absurd to even consider such a request. I argue that passengers would start squirming in their seats if such a thing actually happened. They would think, "Isn't he supposed to be flying the airplane?" Yet, in professional nursing, when the transport department is short of personnel, or the pharmacy does not have enough technicians to run missing drugs to the units, nurses are often expected and required to take on these tasks. The expectation to complete nonnursing functions adds to task saturation, interrupts nursing thought work, and places the patient at risk. We would never expect pilots to sacrifice concentration for the completion of tasks outside the scope of their number one job, which is to fly the airplane. For nurses, their number one job is to assess patients using specialized knowledge and critically think as they expertly manage clinical problems. It therefore seems culturally deficient to allow or require nurses to be pulled off task to complete nonskilled, nonclinical tasks.

Distractions

Earlier we discussed the term "critical flight regime" to describe periods in the cockpit where task load is high and interruptions pose a serious threat to safety. What would be considered a "critical flight regime" for nurses regardless of clinical specialty? Medication administration rapidly comes to mind although there are many others. On the multibed medical surgical unit, nurses spend a significant amount of time engaged in this activity. It is a task that requires thought work and concentration, and it is reasonable for a patient to expect that the completion of this task will not harm them. Yet, medication administration, this "critical regime," is often carried out in an environment replete with noise, distractions, false starts, and interruptions. ◆

◆ Sidebar 1.6

Task interruptions and inadvertent omissions

In *The Principles of Psychiatry*, William James has praised the "the faculty of voluntarily bringing back a wandering attention, over and over again" as the very root of judgment, character, and will. However, in the high-stakes environment of the nursing unit, interruptions, distractions, and unexpected task demands, which impair both individual and team performance, are the norm.[21] Interruptions challenge the cognitive mechanism by which individuals remember to perform intended actions and remember to perform a deferred task. Without an explicit prompt that the time has come to act, it is all too easy to forget.[20] Thus, inadvertent omissions have been shown to constitute the largest class of human performance problems in numerous hazardous operations.[22]

Task completion and focus become difficult as nurses start and stop over and over again. In a sense, the long-standing paradigm in the culture has been that nurses are open season for anyone traversing the unit environment. A few years ago, as a nurse manager on a large medical surgical unit, I, along with an outstanding nursing staff, implemented a CRM-based care delivery model, part of which included mechanisms to reduce distractions modeled after the "sterile cockpit" concept in aviation. A detailed discussion of this implementation, cultural reactions, and relevant literature can be found in Chapter 6.

Standardization

We talked briefly about standardization in the airline culture. In the cockpit, standardization provides a frame of reference, serves to mitigate the unexpected, and allows us to predict behavior in both routine and emergent circumstances. For nurses, it serves the same purpose; however, the clinical environment often falls short in securing adequate levels of standardization. The nursing culture has traditionally been programmed to accommodate varying preferences and idiosyncrasies of physician providers.[15] For example, there are facility-based protocols regarding heparin, sliding scale insulin, and postoperative analgesia, yet some physicians choose to use variations of these protocols based on individual preference. In such cases, nurses are burdened with having to keep tabs on an array of preferences rather than a single standard. This is not optimal from an error avoidance standpoint.

Equipment may differ as well. Defibrillators and hospital beds can vary from unit to unit within the same facility. Vendors can change causing unanticipated changes in syringes and drug packaging. Differences in patient care processes among units can also be commonplace. While some nursing units may be standardized in their processes, their "standards" are not uniform throughout a facility. The result is pockets of differing standardization creating vulnerabilities when nurses are floated (reassigned) from their home unit to unfamiliar clinical areas. Processes that are not standardized institutionally place patients at risk. The case below illustrates this point:

> On 9 North, a medical-surgical unit, the computer generated medication adminis-
> tration record (MAR) schedules a.m. insulin to be given at 0700, which appears
> in the day shift section of the MAR. Although the day shift technically begins at
> 0700, day shift nurses are in report and not available to administer insulin. On
> 9 North, breakfast trays usually arrive right at 0700 as well. Because of this,
> the unit has decided that the night nurse will administer the insulin prior to 0700
> and document on the night shift section of the record.

> 9 East is also a medical-surgical unit. On this unit, the day nurse administers all 0700
> insulin, and it has been done this way for years. One night, a nurse from 9 North is
> floated to 9 East to help with short staffing. Prior to 0700, the nurse administers the
> 0700 insulin as she does on her home unit. This is business as usual to her so she makes
> no mention of this routine activity when she reports to the day shift nurse. The day
> shift nurse on 9 East does not see the night shift documentation of the insulin that was
> given to the patient (there would be no reason for her to check this) and administers
> the a.m. insulin to the patient for the second time, documenting this act in the 0700
> block of the MAR. A few hours later, the patient becomes severely hypoglycemic.

Soaring to Success

Recurrent training and performance checking

When I speak to groups of nurses, I usually ask three questions about recurrent training:

Question 1: Who has practiced in this particular organization for more than 10 years?

Several hands go up.

Question 2: For those that raised their hand, did you attend new employee orientation when you were hired 10 years ago?

Same number of hands goes up.

Question 3: For those that raised their hand, how many have gone back through orientation within those 10 years?

Not a single hand goes up.

It is conceivable that after initial new hire orientation is complete, a nurse will never again return to the classroom setting for a review of basic policy and procedure. They do complete yearly competency or skills check offs, but these are often more of a formality and can be haphazard. Often nurses must complete such check offs on their own time (above and beyond their work schedule), or are expected to squeeze the review into their workday while they are on the unit caring for patients. Usually, this means they will run down to the skills area and move rapidly through multiple stations, completing the yearly requirement in minimum time. Stations are designed for ease of flow rather than detailed practice and challenge. It is not a test of knowledge, but a fulfilling of a requirement: a check off. Completely removing nurses from their clinical duties and sending them to a comfortable learning environment for training and practice, then thoroughly checking performance using high-fidelity simulation is not common practice in the culture. This topic will be outlined further in Chapter 9.

Conclusion

Now the blank page is filled and the culture comparison—aviation on one side and nursing on the other—is complete. I have outlined many areas where professional nursing, in terms of practice and leadership, has much work to do if it is to truly become a culture of safety. Caring and human empathy as a specialty set nursing apart from other disciplines in health-care. This should never be overlooked or lost in any effort to transform the culture. With that said, I steadfastly maintain that the concepts, tools, and practices that define CRM, practices used in cockpits all over the world, provide a sound model for cultural change in professional nursing.

References

1. Starr, P., *The Social Transformation of American Medicine.* 1982, Basic Books: New York.

2. Ozar, D., *Dental Ethics at Chairside.* 2002, Washington, DC: Georgetown University Press.

3. A. Rosenstein, H. Alan, and M. O'Daniel, A Survey of the Impact of Disruptive Behaviors and Communication Defects on Patient Safety. *Joint Commission Journal on Quality and Patient Safety, 2008. 34*(8): p. 464–471.

4. Sine, D.M. and N. Northcutt, Effects of organizational leadership behavior on learning ethics: A study of professional paramedics. *Journal of Emergency Management 2009. 7*(6): p. 61–70.

5. Kotter, J., *Leading Change.* 1996, Boston: Harvard Business School Press.

6. Lewicki, R.L., and B. Bunker, Developing and Maintaining Trust in Work Relationships in *Trust in Organizations: Frontiers of Theory and Research*, R. Kramer and T. Tyler, Editors. 1996, Sage: Thousand Oaks.

7. Woods, D., and R. Cook., Perspectives on Human Error: Hindsight Bias and Local Rationality in *Handbook of Applied Cognition*, F. Durso, R. Nickerson, and J. Schvanevelt, Editors. 1999, Wiley: New York.

8. Casey, S., *Set Phasers on Stun: And Other True Tales of Design, Technology, and Human Error. 1993,* Santa Barbara: Aegean.

9. Bogner, M., *Human Error in Medicine.* 1994, Hillsdale: Lawrence Erlbaum Associates.

10. Rogers, A.E., W.T. Hwang, L.D. Scott, L.H. Aiken, and D.F. Dinges., The working hours of hospital staff nurses and patient safety. *Health Affairs, 2004. 23*(4): p. 202–212.

11. Scott, L.D., A.E. Rogers, W.T. Hwang, and Y. Zhang, Effects of critical care nurses' work hours on vigilance and patients' safety. *American Journal of Critical Care, 2006. 15*(1): p. 30–37.

12. Owens, J.A., Sleep Loss and Fatigue in Healthcare Professionals. *Journal of Perinatal and Neonatal Nursing, 2007 21*(2): p. 91–100.

13. Aiken, L.H., S.P. Clarke, D.M. Sloane, J. Sochalski, and J.H. Silber, Hospital nurse staffing and patient mortality, nurse burnout, and job dissatisfaction. *JAMA, 2002. 288*(16): p. 1987–1993.

14. Sine, D. and G. Sculli, Just Checking: Using Team Briefings to Improve Patient Safety. *Healthbeat, 2010. 9*(3): p. 4–6.

15. Nemeth, C., *Improving Healthcare Team Communication: Building on Lessons from Aviation and Aerospace.* 2009, Burlington: Ashgate.

16. Miller, J., *Controlling Pilot Error: Fatigue.* 2001, New York: McGraw Hill.

17. Rosen, C., The Myth of Multitasking. *The New Atlantis,* 2008. Spring 2008(20): p. 105–110.

18. Poldrack, R. *How Multitasking Affects Human Learning.* 2007 [cited 7/13/2010]; Available from: *www.npr.org/templates/story/story.php?storyId=7700581.*

19. Gleick, J., *Faster: The Acceleration of Just About Everything.* 1999, New York: Pantheon.

20. Loukopoulos, L., R. Dismukes, and I. Barshi, *The Multitaskng Myth.* 2009, Burlington: Ashgate.

21. Pape, T.M., Applying airline safety pratices to medication administration. *Medsurg Nursing, 2003. 12*(2): p. 77–93.

22. Reason, J., Combating omission errors through task analysis and good reminders. *Quality and Safety in Health Care, 2002. 11*: p. 40–44.

Soaring to Success

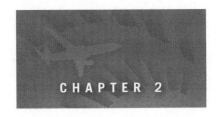

What Is Crew Resource Management?

Tragedy Prompted Development of Crew Resource Management

This book is about nursing, but I will ask you as the reader to indulge me for a moment. I would like to take you back in time and analyze two classic airline disasters that are central to the genesis of crew resource management (CRM). Understanding these airline errors will enrich your understanding of further discussions on the topic. This chapter will briefly discuss what CRM is, where it came from, and what it aims to achieve. Finally, it will outline salient CRM topics and concepts that can be applied to nursing practice. Many of these concepts will be expanded upon throughout the book.

Tenerife

On March 27, 1977, two Boeing passenger jets collided on the runway at Los Rodeos Airport located on the Spanish island of Tenerife, one of the Canary Islands. At one end of the runway, a Pan American 747 taxiing slowly ahead was to exit the runway at an upcoming turnoff. At the opposite end of the same runway, the crew of the other Boeing jet, a Dutch KLM 747, sat waiting for the Pan American aircraft to clear the runway so it could begin its takeoff roll. To complicate matters, the airport was enshrouded in mist and fog that greatly reduced visibility. Strangely enough, neither aircraft was supposed to be at Los Rodeos that day. Because a bomb had exploded at their original destination of Los Palmas Airport on the nearby island of Gran Canaria, both flights were diverted to Tenerife until it was deemed safe to continue.

While the Pan American crew continued their taxi in the mist, searching for the turnoff, the Dutch captain, increasingly concerned about exceeding duty time regulations, grew ever more impatient with the delays. Suddenly, he pushed the throttles of the KLM jumbo jet forward, beginning its acceleration down the runway. Moments later, the Pan American crew spotted the lights of the KLM airliner barreling down on them. They desperately tried to clear the runway, the pilots exclaiming, "Get off! Get off! Get off!" The KLM jet, just barely airborne and gaining speed, collided with the Pan Am as it was turning off the runway. Both aircraft burst into flames. The KLM's momentum carried it forward, where it crashed out of control, disintegrating and burning. The Pan American sat helpless, with much of the aircraft destroyed and engulfed in a massive inferno. Of the 644 passengers and crew on both aircraft, there were 583 fatalities, 48 of whom were children. Only 61 people survived. It was a disaster of enormous magnitude. It was later determined that the KLM captain, in his haste, initiated the takeoff without receiving clearance from the control tower—a disastrous move.[1]

Linguistic analyses of conversations in the KLM cockpit revealed an insidious communication pattern among the crew. Both the first officer and flight engineer were clearly intimidated by the captain's authoritative style and status. This led them to assume an overly subordinate behavioral mode in much of their interactions with the captain, right up to the moment of the crash.[2] When the captain began the takeoff without proper clearance, neither the copilot nor flight engineer challenged him, despite their apprehension and unease with his actions. At one point early in the takeoff, with the aircraft gaining speed, the flight engineer raised his concern about the possibility of a collision, but the feedback was presented as a question rather than a direct statement, and thus was easily dismissed by the captain. This exchange is presented below:

> *Flight engineer: Is hijerneitaf-dan?. (Is he not clear, then?)*
> *Captain: Watzag je? (What did you say?)*
> *Flight engineer: Is hijernietaf die Pan American? (Is he not clear, that Pan American?)*
> *Captain: Jawal (Yes [with emphasis].)*

Thirteen seconds later, the two jets collided.

UAL Portland

Fast-forward one year to 1978. United Airlines Flight 173 departed Denver, CO, for its destination of Portland, OR. When configuring for the approach at Portland, the crew experienced a malfunction with the landing gear, so they circled close to the airport and went to work correcting the problem.[3] While they had cause to believe the wheels were down and locked, they could not be certain, so the captain continued to circle and began discussing emergency landing procedures with the lead flight attendant. He then informed his cockpit crew, a copilot and flight engineer, that he expected to remain aloft for another 15 minutes before landing. Hearing this, the two crew members became very concerned that there wasn't enough fuel remaining to stay aloft that long. Below is an excerpt from the transcript of cockpit crew conversation after the captain declares that he will be delaying the landing another 15 minutes:

> *First officer responds: Fifteen minutes?*
> *Captain responds: Yeah ...*
> *Flight engineer responds: Not enough. Fifteen minutes is gonna really run us low on fuel here.*

This is a critical moment for Flight 173. The captain offers no response to the terse question posed by the first officer and does not acknowledge the warning from the flight

Soaring to Success

engineer. He simply is not engaged in the sense of urgency felt by his team. Moments later, the flight engineer again attempts to warn the captain that the fuel quantity is reaching a critical point:

> **Flight engineer warns:** *We got about three on the fuel and that's it. (Means 3,000 pounds)*

The captain again does not acknowledge the flight engineer's warning.

Just as in the Tenerife case, both crew members assumed an overly subordinate posture, never confronting the captain's decision head on, never demanding or requiring that he respond. Instead of asserting their concerns directly and gaining resolution toward a different course of action, the crew depends on cautious suggestion as their method to convey what they are certain is a perilous situation. Moments later, each of the four engines on the jetliner began failing, one by one. The aircraft went down in darkness about six miles from the airport in a wooded section of residential Portland. Miraculously, 179 passengers survived, but 24 were seriously injured. Ten people were fatally injured, including the flight engineer.

What happened?

The Dutch 747 involved in the Tenerife accident was flown by none other than KLM's chief instructor pilot. He had logged more than 11,000 flight hours and was a well-known and highly respected senior captain at the airline. The Pan American crew totaled more than 47,000 hours between the three pilots. The United Airlines jet in the Portland crash was piloted by a captain who had more than 27,000 hours of flying time. The entire United crew combined had more than 36,000 hours in the air, and each crew member had successfully completed all recent proficiency checks.

How could this have happened? How is it possible that experienced, expert pilots—who were at the top of their profession—deemed technically competent, could be involved in such drastically fatal and seemingly preventable mishaps? Why would captains not solicit input from the rest of the team when making decisions? Why would other members of the crew sit by and not assert their concerns, even in the face of impending disaster? These questions can be answered with one word: **culture**.

Three decades ago, airline culture was much different than it is today. At that time the culture placed great emphasis on the captain's individual authority, not on teamwork. The captain had supreme rule and subordinate crew members did not question actions and decisions freely, nor were they actively encouraged to do so. Pilot training emphasized technical flying skill above all else, and it was thought that a technically competent pilot, coupled with adherence to procedure, was sufficient to achieve acceptable levels of operational safety. Clearly, these two accidents provide incontrovertible evidence to the contrary. Technical prowess, knowledge, experience, and superb hand-eye coordination were not enough.

Human beings are vulnerable to many environmental and psychological forces that can degrade the integrity of decisions, especially in complex situations. This helps explain why the KLM captain became consumed with his efforts to beat the clock and continued with a course of action that, at face value, seemed counter to reason and safety. It explains why the United captain continued to delay landing while failing to address or acknowledge the aircraft's fuel status. It therefore makes sense that industries that carry out safety-sensitive endeavors with little margin for error, must embrace a cultural paradigm that recognizes the **fallibility of decision makers, the dangers of rigid authority, and the need for open communication and teamwork as a countermeasure**.

CRM: The Beginning

The National Aeronautics and Space Administration (NASA) began addressing the issue in the late 1970s. In 1979, NASA sponsored a workshop entitled "Resource Management on the Flight Deck." The workshop presented research that demonstrated that the majority of air transport accidents were occurring not because of mechanical failures, but because of human failures: failures in decision making, failures in leadership, and failures in inter-personal communications among flight crews.[4] In other words, what happened at Tenerife and Portland was a common theme emerging in postaccident analysis all over the world. Someone on the team knew that something bad was about to happen, but anomalies in the professional culture made it difficult, if not impossible, to speak up forcefully enough to change the outcome.

Representatives from several air carriers attended and came away from the experience with a commitment to develop and implement CRM training programs at their respective airlines. The stated purpose of CRM was to reduce error through the better use of the human resources on the flight deck. The training programs aimed to enhance the "interpersonal aspects of flight." This is an important statement because this training represented an entirely different focus that meant moving away from previously held cultural norms that drove cockpit behavior and communication. Initial programs advocated a departure from **autocratic and overly authoritative** styles of aircraft command, promoting participatory leadership styles that acknowledge the importance of an interdependent team. Equally important was the focus on methods to increase involvement and assertiveness on the part of subordinate crew members when safety was in question.[4, 5]

CRM continues on

Think back to a time in nursing when a new initiative was started in a department or on a unit. No doubt you witnessed significant pushback from naysayers and those who were naturally resistant to change. The airlines experienced similar reactions to early CRM training. Some pilots, for example, described the experience as "charm school" and "psycho-babble" and resisted its premise. The majority of pilots, however, found great value in the training. Rather than fade away, CRM programs took hold and continued to evolve over the next several decades.[4, 6]

In nursing, when new practice initiatives encounter turbulence they often die off, slowly losing momentum, then disappearing from the radar as other priorities take hold. Why did

CRM in the airlines not experience the same fate? The answer lies in steadfast industry and organizational leadership.

What is impressive about the advent of CRM in commercial aviation is that airlines were ready and willing to address failures in the existing professional culture before they were mandated to do so by federal agencies.[5] Top airline managers didn't reject the idea exclaiming, "We can't implement this without more data," "We don't know if it will work," or "It's not evidence-based," all phrases heard frequently in healthcare. It was implemented because it made sense and because the stakes were high.

CRM was able to continue and evolve because airline leaders understood that culture change is a marathon, not a sprint. They committed resources to it and didn't take their eye off the ball. To put it bluntly, CRM wasn't offered as an option; it was mandated. Strident resistors were not appeased. Pilots were required to assimilate and standardize CRM behaviors in the interest of safety. If not, there was always the option to seek employment elsewhere. A critical ingredient in sustaining CRM in the airline industry is the performance evaluation or "check ride" discussed in Chapter 1. These Federal Aviation Administration-mandated events take place in aircraft simulators at regular intervals and allow airline instructors to reinforce and grade pilots on adherence to CRM behaviors. Airline leaders mandated it from the top down, but it was the simulation events that buttressed it from the bottom up. ◆

◆ Sidebar 2.1

A sustainable critical mass

When new ideas or technologies are introduced, there will always be some resistance. If a change is to be truly transformative, the visible behaviors must become the everyday assumptions of the group that eventually become less apparent but deeply ingrained shared values. Must there be a minimum number of believers in the group who are committed to the change? Business leadership consultants assert that between 12% and 15% of a group must commit to the new concepts before a significant change can occur. If the change is to be sustained, and a regression to the familiar avoided, a majority of group members, and virtually all of leadership, must believe the change is essential.[7, 8]

As is the case with cultural change, many resistors eventually retired and those pilots who grew up with CRM became captains, managers, and flight instructors. In due course, life on the flight deck was transformed.

CRM: Today

Since the original programs of the 1980s, CRM training has evolved to include additional subject matter beyond a focus on interpersonal communication. Today CRM core content typically includes topics such as leadership, team building, followership and conflict resolution, decision making, human factors, situational awareness, and managing automation and technology.[4, 9, 10] Today, at many airlines, CRM appears less as a stand-alone program, and instead has seen its concepts become firmly entrenched in all facets of airline training. Specific behaviors have been embedded and standardized in day-to-day operations. For example, pilots provide verbal readbacks and callouts to each other before moving or selecting critical switches in the cockpit; formal briefings at key points during a flight appear as specific items to be completed on cockpit checklists. **CRM is not a seminar or class; it's a way of life.**

Think of it this way: CRM has two main parts. The first deals with **teamwork and communication** and covers the interpersonal and social aspects of the working environment. The second deals with **human factors and situational awareness** and entails understanding physical and cognitive limitations, while outlining strategies to manage elements in the operational environment such as fatigue, high task load, distractions, and automation. Although there are many topics that descend from these two broad categories, for me it is a straightforward way to organize the basics of CRM.

The goal of CRM and how it relates to nursing

As previously stated, the goal of CRM is to reduce error, and at face value this is a noble cause that makes sense. However, another more recent view regarding the objective of CRM is the idea of error management. This view moves away from the goal of reducing and/or eliminating error (e.g., zero tolerance) and shifts the premise of CRM to detecting and lessening the effects of error.[11, 12] A fundamental principle with the concept of error management is that human error is inevitable; it is going to happen whether we like it or not, so why not apply CRM tools as a set of countermeasures to discover and control errors before they escalate into mishaps and catastrophic events. Figure 2.1 is a model that explains the error management process, which has three steps: avoidance, trapping, and mitigation. To illustrate, let's use a nursing scenario and apply the error management pyramid.

FIGURE
2.1

Error Management Pyramid

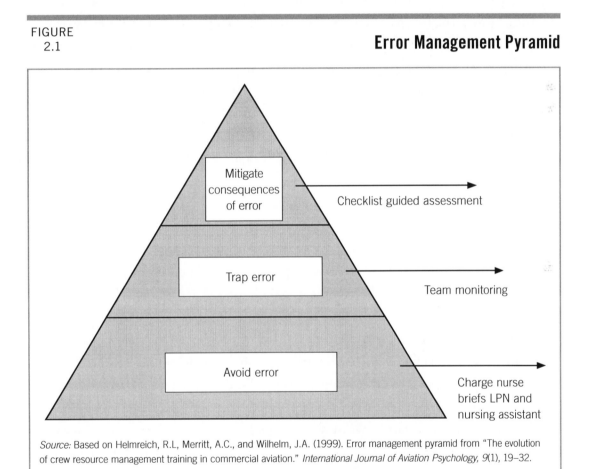

Source: Based on Helmreich, R.L, Merritt, A.C., and Wilhelm, J.A. (1999). Error management pyramid from "The evolution of crew resource management training in commercial aviation." *International Journal of Aviation Psychology, 9*(1), 19–32.

The bottom of the pyramid is where we implement CRM strategies to avoid error. For example, a charge nurse on a med-surg unit takes a moment to brief a licensed practical nurse (LPN) and nursing assistant that several patients will be returning from surgery in a compressed time frame. She reviews postoperative assessment protocol, discusses workload planning, and reinforces the need to promptly speak up to the rest of the team if problems or abnormalities arise.

This should assist in the avoidance of errors in postoperative patient care. The next step in the pyramid is error trapping. This means that an error has already been made, but CRM strategies detect and "trap," or stop, the error from reaching the patient. An example in our scenario would be the charge nurse actively monitoring the actions of team members as they care for newly received postoperative patients. In doing so, she notices that the LPN has become sidetracked in assisting another patient and is not conducting patient assessments at a frequency required by protocol. The charge nurse attends to the postoperative patient and promptly discovers tachycardia and a marked drop in blood pressure. She notifies the LPN and together they manage the patient. The LPN became distracted and did not maintain postoperative monitoring; in this sense an error has already occurred. Team monitoring (discussed in Chapter 8) traps this error and stops it from progressing to the point where the patient experiences continued unnoticed decline.

The final step is error mitigation. Let's now suppose that neither a team briefing nor team monitoring is successful in avoiding or trapping the error. When the LPN finally finishes tending to her other patient, she realizes that time has gotten away from her and it's been too long since she has assessed the postop patient in her care. She enters the patient's room and immediately sees that his condition is not stable, but she is not sure what is going on. She notifies the charge nurse and then references a checklist that the unit developed to assist in the assessment and management of unstable patients. The checklist guides the team's assessment step by step. Soon it is verified that the patient has unstable vital signs, pallor, and frank bleeding at the operative site. The checklist then guides the team to increase IV fluids, apply oxygen, and call the rapid response team. In short time, the patient is transferred off unit. Again, the error has occurred; the patient was not monitored as closely or as frequently as required. Unfortunately, this patient was experiencing active bleeding and although it was not discovered sooner, a checklist-guided assessment assured accurate clinical responses with little time wasted. The effect of the initial error on the patient was mitigated.

It is important to remember that error management is not a blame game. The premise is that any professional (nurses, pilots, etc.) will make mistakes, not because of individual failures that must be remediated, but because we as human beings have performance limitations that will occasionally fall short of what the operational environment demands. Therefore, we look at CRM strategies as a safety net to trap and minimize the effect of the errors we are bound to make before they result in harm and injury. This premise is completely consistent with a systems-based nonpunitive response to error and is consistent with efforts to increase event reporting among nursing staff. In my view, presenting CRM within the context of error management offers a profoundly strong case for the rapid acceptance and implementation of CRM programs in nursing practice. ◆

◆ Sidebar 2.2

Making sense of things

Teams extract cues from their environmental context to help them decide what information is relevant and what explanations of conditions are acceptable to maintain high-quality care and patient safety. These small cues, which often take the form of simple familiar structures, are used to develop a bigger picture of what is happening to a patient.[13, 14] Team members construct, rearrange, single out, and reject objective information to create a subjective abstraction of reality and make sense of their environment.[15] Sense for a team is created through conversation and the give-and-take of dialogue as teams move ideas around to reach a shared understanding of what is happening, what is possible, and what is probable.

CRM Works—But Can We Prove It?

I want to state categorically that CRM reduces risk and enhances safety in high-risk operations. As an airline pilot, I lived and practiced CRM on a daily basis both as a captain and as a copilot. I can easily recall multiple times where specific communication techniques and/or situational awareness strategies trapped errors and sorted out confusion before it became a bigger problem. I have also seen it produce positive results on nursing units at the point of care (more on this later).

It is generally accepted that fatal accidents occur so infrequently at the airlines that fatality rates cannot be used to provide statistically significant evidence for the effect of CRM programs.[4, 9, 12] However, when airline fatal events are examined globally over time, interesting interpretations emerge. Steve Lambrecht is a Navy Top Gun graduate, former airline pilot, and managing partner of Mach 1 Solutions, a company that conducts CRM training for medical teams. Lambrecht looked at global fatal events per million flights from 1970–2004 (see Figure 2.2) and offers the following interpretation: From 1970, the fatal accident rate decreased sharply until it leveled out in the early 1980s. This is mainly due to advances in technology: better autopilot, navigation, and warning systems.

FIGURE
2.2

Result of CRM in Aviation

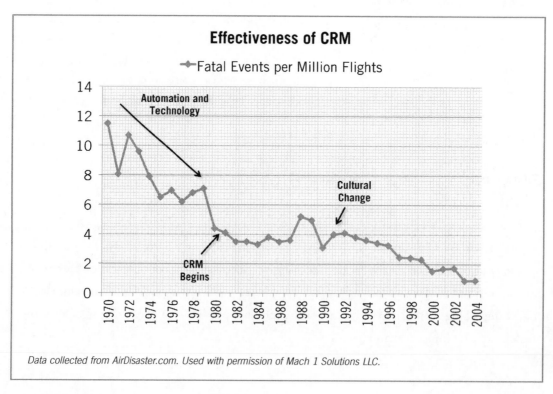

Data collected from AirDisaster.com. Used with permission of Mach 1 Solutions LLC.

Throughout the early 1980s, the rate is relatively stable with peaks and valleys occurring in the later part of the decade. Then it gets interesting in the early 1990s. At this time, we see a steady and measured dropoff in the global fatal event rate until it bottoms out and stabilizes around 2003 to its lowest point over the 34-year period.

So, what happened? United Airlines implemented the first CRM program in 1981. As we just discussed, the training took hold, evolved, and became embedded in all aspects of airline operations. The marked and steady dropoff in the early 1990s occurred after CRM had 10 full years to permeate the industry. At this point, we see the effects of true cultural change as CRM behaviors that support communication, teamwork, and situational awareness are manifested. In this context, examining rates provides a persuasive argument for the effectiveness of CRM.

A more recognized metric for the validation of CRM concepts lies in human responses to the training. Empirical studies across high-risk industries and other aviation specific data, demonstrate that CRM training produces large positive changes in both operational behaviors as well as attitudes about safety.

This applies to airlines, military flight operations, nuclear power, offshore drilling, and healthcare.[4, 6, 9] With that said, let's briefly focus on healthcare, an industry that unfortunately cannot currently demonstrate the level of safety found in the other high-risk industries mentioned.

CRM in Healthcare and Nursing

Elements of CRM have been taught and applied in healthcare settings to improve teamwork and communication. For example:

- Within the Veterans Administration, a Medical Team Training Program teaches the use of briefings among surgery teams. Statistically significant improvements were observed in team communication scores, timeliness of preoperative antibiotics, timeliness of deep vein thrombosis prophylaxis, and perioperative mortality.[16, 17]

- A global study by the World Health Organization demonstrated statistically significant reductions in postoperative mortality and complications with the use of a surgical safety checklist.[18]

- CRM training was implemented over one year in a multidisciplinary obstetrical setting. Participants demonstrated a significant positive change in their knowledge of teamwork and shared decision making. Positive changes were noted in the teamwork, safety climate, and stress recognition dimensions of a safety attitude assessment.

- A CRM-based human factors training program was administered in surgery departments at five facilities across the United States. Core CRM concepts and tools were implemented. A patient safety culture survey was administered to staff pre- and post-training throughout the five hospitals (n = 688). Collectively, participants had an average 7.4% increase in all 12 dimensions of the survey. The largest gains occurred in the dimensions measuring teamwork, handoffs, and event reporting.[19]

- An aviation-based team training program was taught to patients at Dana Farber Cancer Institute, covering briefings, assertive communication, closed loop communication, and situational awareness. Thirty-nine percent of patients reported a change in their behavior regarding the level of involvement in their care.[20]

CRM initiatives are producing positive changes worldwide in the knowledge, behavior, and attitudes of healthcare teams, along with measurable improvement in clinical outcomes. So, let's build on this momentum! The 2004 Institute of Medicine report entitled *Keeping Patients Safe: Transforming the Work Environment for Nurses* emphasizes that nurses are the largest contingent of clinical providers, and they play a critical role in the surveillance and rescue of patients. Allocating resources to implement and sustain a comprehensive CRM training program tailored specifically for nursing units is a warranted and logical next step. ◆

CRM Concepts Applied to Nursing

What I said in the preface of the book is worth repeating here: Simply dropping CRM into professional nursing will not work. Nurses are not pilots, and patients are not airplanes. CRM concepts must first be modified to fit the unique nursing practice environment if they are to be accepted and applied in a lasting fashion. Figure 2.3 is a chart that identifies salient CRM concepts with a brief description of their application to clinical practice.

◆ Sidebar 2.3
A power distance culture

One of the dimensions of organizational and national culture described by Geert Hofstede is "power distance," the degree to which power is distributed unequally among group members. In large power distance organizational cultures, members without power are unlikely to approach or question leaders and accept that power is distributed unequally. Typically, those in charge have a monopoly on the decision-making process. In small power distance cultures, subordinates are less apt to depend on leaders and are comfortable contributing to and even questioning decisions by those in power.[21-23]

When CRM aviation programs were first exported from the United States to other countries, problems emerged in large power distance cultures. In China and Latin American countries, where subordinates accept power relations that are paternalistic or autocratic, the tenets of CRM—speaking up, asserting concerns, and questioning decisions—were not well received.[24]

Therefore, a common recommendation prior to implementing CRM training in any industry is to assess the power distance of the existing culture first. For teams that exist on nursing units, an excellent question to ask is "Is our prevailing organizational culture large or small power distance?" This question has great relevance, particularly with respect to the us/them boundary in the nurse/physician dyad, which has historically been a source of great friction.[25, 26] For a nurse leader, power distance can also be used to identify beliefs and social structures that may be obstacles to the adoption of CRM and what part of CRM—teamwork and communication or humans factors and situation awareness—will require the greater emphasis during implementation.

FIGURE
2.3

Applying CRM to Clinical Practice

CRM Concept	Application to nursing
Leadership styles and teambuilding	Nurses are leaders on their units and practice in teams that take on various forms. It is imperative that nurses apply leadership styles that encourage open communication and inquiry from other team members, especially when patient safety is in question. Nurses implement specific strategies and behaviors that facilitate teamwork and the timely exchange of relevant clinical information among staff.
Situational awareness	Situational awareness (SA) can be thought of as the ability to perceive what is occurring in the environment, the prioritization and attachment of meaning to what is perceived to form a clinical picture, and the projection of what will happen in the near future. SA is the precursor to decision making and is expressed as being high or low. Higher levels of SA are associated with decision making that is both sound and safe. Nurses practice in a complex, dynamic, and safety sensitive environment where higher levels of SA are required. Nurses benefit from understanding the forces in their environment that threaten SA, as well as knowing how to recognize circumstances where clinical SA is at risk, and what to do to maintain it. Through the implementation of processes such as actively monitoring team members for the effects of task saturation and fatigue, along with the use of tools like checklists and briefings, nurses can preserve higher levels of SA to support clinical decision making.
Followership: Assertive inquiry and advocacy	In addition to being leaders on their units, nurses also assume supportive roles on patient care teams. Registered nurses support physicians who are the leader of the medical team and the final authority for decisions regarding a patient's medical treatment plan. Nurses spend the majority of the time with patients who are hospitalized. It is imperative, therefore, that nurses, in addition to practicing effective leadership, also practice followership. Followership is an active role that demands critical thinking and an ability to communicate concerns about patient safety directly and promptly. Nurses as effective followers practice inquiry (questioning patient care decisions) and advocacy (promoting an alternate course of action deemed to be safer than what is planned) regardless of rank or stature in the organization. Well-executed followership is also pivotal in a nurse's ability to formulate assertive statements, and to resolve conflicts about patient care decisions.
Workload management	Division of work, especially during periods of high task and mental load, can reduce cognitive demand, allowing for higher SA and better decision making. Nurses can divide up routine patient care functions such as patient assessments, admitting, and medication administration as an example. Workload management encompasses effective delegation by nurse team leaders, especially during emergency situations. It also includes knowing and utilizing "all available resources" at their disposal in order to manage workload. Leadership is an integral part of effective workload management.

FIGURE
2.3

Applying CRM to Clinical Practice *(cont.)*

CRM Concept	Application to nursing
Managing automation and technology	Automation and technology is prevalent in the clinical environment. While automation can reduce workload and allow for continuous monitoring of patient status, it can reduce a nurses SA. Precepts regarding technology management center on: • Not having implicit trust in the ability of automation to always function correctly in monitoring • Maintaining vigilance and adhering to policies, procedures, and standards when working with automation • Not allowing technology and automation to deplete or replace basic clinical assessment skills • Cross-checking automated information with what is actually seen (raw patient assessment data) and resolving discrepancies
Reducing distractions during critical tasks	Nurses implement specific changes on the unit designed to reduce interruptions and distractions during critical tasks or time periods. Implementations can include the use of protected zones in medication preparation areas, the use of vests and other discernable indicators, and signage. Mechanisms to protect nurses from distractions can also include physical alterations to the unit layout as well as protocol changes that serve to reduce noise and traffic. This concept is based on the airline's "sterile cockpit" rule that protects pilots from distractions, and prohibits pilots from engaging in behavior that diverts attention.
Fatigue awareness	Fatigue reduces SA and is a significant threat to clinical performance and decision making. Nurses can frequently discuss fatigue awareness in unit briefings, monitor each other for signs of fatigue, and implement operational countermeasures to manage its effects. Sanctioning short naps during extended shifts is one example of a fatigue countermeasure.
Verifying actions and inputs	Nurses use redundancy and double checks with another staff member to verify critical actions and inputs. Situations on the unit where this may occur are: programming infusion pumps; changing ventilator settings; administering high risk medications; or administering chemotherapy. The verification is not passive agreement or formality, but true double checks where both staff members are fully engaged in the clinical scenario.

Soaring to Success

FIGURE
2.3

Applying CRM to Clinical Practice *(cont.)*

CRM Concept	Application to nursing
Checklists	Checklists are used to support memory in both routine and emergent situations. With routine tasks, nurses can develop and use checklists to verify that steps are not missed as a result of distractions and interruptions. In emergent situations nurses can use checklists to guide the decision-making process and support SA.
Briefings	Briefings enhance teamwork and communication. Briefings also support team SA. Nurse team leaders use structured briefings to communicate pertinent patient information, team behavioral expectations, goals, and areas for focused patient assessment. The briefing is also used as an opportunity to have controlled team discussion to clarify questions and address concerns. Briefings can occur, for example, between a registered nurse and a nursing assistant working together during a shift, or be conducted as a safety briefing led by the unit charge nurse for all staff before the start of a shift. Briefings can also be used prior to a procedure or treatment on the unit.
Debriefings	Debriefings are structured discussions facilitated by a team leader for the purposes of reviewing individual and team performance in an open blame free atmosphere. The Debriefing serves to identify areas where the team performed well along with areas for improvement, and serves to build teamwork, communication and SA for future challenges. Debriefings can be applied after routine events but should be used after emergent or adverse occurrences. For example: Nurse team leaders can conduct debriefings after a code, fall with injury or significant patient complaint
Error management	Human error is inevitable. The focus therefore is not to eliminate error, but rather to develop methods and countermeasures to mitigate its effect on the system. Mechanisms can be applied to avoid, trap or reduce the effects of human error; this is called placing "fault tolerance" in a system. Rather than seeing themselves as individuals functioning independently of a system that delivers care, nurses move to a paradigm that examines their interactions with other people and disciplines as part of a system. It is here where nurses look beyond their own actions, and examine the vulnerabilities that arise from these interactions. Nurses identify vulnerabilities and develop unit based countermeasures to manage error and reduce patient harm.

FIGURE
2.3

Applying CRM to Clinical Practice *(cont.)*

CRM Concept	Application to nursing
Standardization	Standardization: • Is necessary to ensure that policies and procedures will be followed regardless of individual personalities or beliefs • Allows professionals to know and execute learned procedures which reduce cognitive load on attention and working memory • Allows professionals to predict the actions and behaviors of others in a given circumstance. • Nurses can use standardization to optimize performance and SA between shifts and between units. Nurses can also use standardization to detect the effects of staff fatigue, task overload, or incapacitation—all of which can lead to error. For example: If a nurse is deviating from standard procedure or behaving in a manner that is not consistent with protocol, this can be detected by other staff members and resolved before it reaches the patient.
Recurrent training and competency practice	A hallmark of high-reliability organizations is ongoing training and practice via the use of simulation. Recurrent training ensures that professionals revisit important policies, standards and operating procedures at specified intervals. Competency practice using simulation ensures that professionals can safely practice dealing with infrequent clinical situations in a safe environment. Over time, book knowledge can fade, the rationale for routine actions is not remembered, and fresh knowledge is replaced by the realities of day-to-day operations. Ultimately complacency can set in and the ability to respond accurately and timely in an emergent or abnormal situation decays. Nurses can implement a recurrent training and competency practice model. The model allows nurses to immerse themselves in training that takes place in an appropriate learning environment, occurs away from the unit, and is free of the pressures of patient assignments. The program occurs at 12-month intervals and consists of a classroom session, which revisits relevant clinical policies and procedures, and a competency practice session, which uses human patient simulation. Classroom and simulation sessions at regular intervals for front-line nursing staff reinforces standardization, reduces complacency, and enhances SA.

Soaring to Success

References

1. Air Safety Network. Flight Safety Report 1977 0327. [cited 2010 11/12/2010]; Available from: *http://aviation-safety.net/database/record.php?id=19770327-1*.

2. McCreary, J., et al., Human factors: Tenerife revisited. *Journal of Air Transportation World Wide, 1998. 3*(1).

3. National Transportation Safety Board, United Air Lines, Inc. McDonnel-Douglas DC-8-61, N8082U Portland, OR: December 28, 1978. 1978.

4. Helmreich, R.L., A.C. Merritt, and J.A. Wilhelm, The evolution of crew resource management training in commercial aviation. *International Journal of Aviation Psychology, 1999. 9*(1): p. 19–32.

5. Musson, D.M. and R.L. Helmreich, Team training and resource management in health care: Current issues and future directions. *Harvard Health Policy Review, 2004. 5*(1): p. 25–35.

6. Helmreich, R. and J. Wilhelm, Outcomes of crew resource management training. *International Journal of Aviation Psychology, 1991. 1*(4): p. 287–300.

7. Kotter, J., *Leading Change.* 1996, Boston: Harvard Business School Press.

8. Gladwell, M., *The Tipping Point: How Little Things Can Make a Big Difference.* 2000, New York: Little, Brown, and Company.

9. O'Connor, P., et al., Crew resource management training effectiveness: A meta-analysis and some critical needs. *International Journal of Aviation Psychology, 2008. 18*(4): p. 353–368.

10. FAA, Crew Resource Management Training AC 120-51E. 2004, U.S. Department of Transportation.

11. Helmreich, R., A.C. Merritt, and J.A. Wilhelm, The Evolution of Crew Resource Management Training in Commercial Aviation. *International Journal of Aviation Psychology, 2008. 9*(1): p. 19–32.

12. Kern, A.T., *Controlling Pilot Error: Culture, Environment, & CRM.* 2001, New York: McGraw Hill. p. 75–77.

13. Weick, K., *Sensemaking in Organizations.* 1995, Thousand Oaks, CA: Sage.

14. Klein, G., *Sources of Power: How People Make Decisions.* 1999, Cambridge, MA: MIT Press.

15. Weick, K., *The Social Psychology of Organizing.* 1979, New York: McGraw-Hill.

16. Awad, S., et al., Bridging the communication gap in the operating room with medical team training. *The American Journal of Surgery 2005. 190*: p. 770–774.

17. Neily, J., et al., Association Between Implementation of a Medical Team Training Program and Surgical Mortality. *JAMA, October 20, 2010; 304*: p. 1693–1700., 2010: p. 1693–1700.

18. Haynes, A., et al., A surgical safety checklist to reduce morbidity and mortality in a global population. *New England Journal of Medicine, 2009. 360*: p. 491–9.

19. Marshall, D.A. and D.A. Manus, A team training program using human factors to enhance patient safety. *AORN Journal, 2007. 86*(6): p. 994–1011.

20. Weingart, S., et al., The You CAN Campaign: Teamwork Training for Patients and Families in Ambulatory Oncology. *Joint Commission Journal on Quality and Patient Safety, 2009. 35*(2): p. 63–71.

21. Hofstede, G., Culture's Consequences: comparing values, behaviors, institutions and organizations across nations. 2 ed. 2001, Thousand Oaks, CA: Sage.

22. Northcutt, N. and D. McCoy, *Interactive Qualitative Analysis.* 2004, Thousand Oaks, CA: Sage.

23. Hofstede, G., Motivation, leadership, and organization: Do American theories apply abroad? *Organizational Dynamics*, 1980(Summer): p. 42–63.

24. Helmreich, R. and A.C. Merritt, *Culture at work in aviation and medicine: National, organizational, and professional influences* 1998, Aldershot, UK: Ashgate.

25. Tilly, C., *Credit and Blame.* 2008, Princeton, NJ: Princeton University Press.

26. Bosk, C.L., *Forgive and Remember.* 1979, Chicago: University of Chicago Press.

Soaring to Success

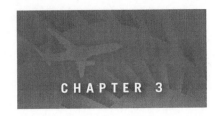

CHAPTER 3

Behave Like a Leader: Value Your Team

LEARNING OBJECTIVES

After reading this chapter, the participant will be able to:

- Describe the effect of poor leadership on team effectiveness

- Identify the characteristics of good leadership

- Discuss strategies for improving teamwork

In Chapter 2, we defined crew resource management (CRM) and discussed its origins, emphasizing that the need for CRM arose from linking poor operational outcomes to teamwork and communication failures. It is important, however, to make the point that any CRM tool adopted with the intent to enhance team effectiveness, such as briefings, checklists, and standardized communication, will ultimately fail without high-quality leadership driving the process. Effective leadership is a central tenet of CRM, with all things descending from there.

In this chapter we will look at a few examples of leader behavior, some good, some not so good. We will also discuss general traits and attitudes found in leaders who are said to practice "good CRM."

Where's The Team, Dr. Bill?

I was a nurse manager on a 40-bed medical–surgical unit. One day, as I often did, I decided to make rounds on the unit to talk with the staff and visit patients. As I walked down a long hall that made up half of the unit, I saw the usual sights: patients ambulating while steadily rolling their IV poles, the busy multidisciplinary activity at the nurses' station, nurses moving in and out of patient rooms, and medication carts parked neatly against the wall.

As I reached the end of the hall, I noticed a nurse, whom I will refer to as Beth, talking on the phone. From her tone and facial expressions, I could tell Beth was frustrated. As I listened, I heard Beth say, "Well, I know that you just saw him, but I'm telling you what I'm finding here. I think it's important and I thought you would want to know." I would later learn that on the other end of the phone the patient's surgeon simply said, "I'll be up" and then hung up the phone.

I asked Beth what was going on and she explained. Beth had an elderly patient with severe peripheral vascular disease who had just returned from surgery to restore blood flow to the lower extremities. As she conducted her postoperative assessment, Beth noticed that the IV in the patient's left forearm was not running correctly. The site looked red and swollen, and the infusion pump was beginning to indicate an occlusion. As she continued her assessment, Beth also noticed that the patient's left hand looked blanched; there was poor capillary refill, and she could not obtain a peripheral radial pulse, even with a Doppler. The patient was also complaining that his hand felt numb. Beth was concerned about getting an IV restarted in the patient but was not comfortable proceeding in that arm. She felt she needed to notify the surgeon right away regarding the apparent lack of circulation in the left arm and hand. When she did so, the surgeon said to her, "I just saw him in recovery. He was fine there." This is where I walked up and heard Beth's response on the phone.

After going in the room with Beth to review her findings, we went back into the hallway. I complimented her on her astute assessment and solid judgment in calling the physician to relay her concerns. What happened next was astonishing. As we stood by her medication cart discussing the issue at hand, the surgeon, whom I'll call Dr. Bill, came walking down the hall looking straight ahead. In tow was a female nurse dressed in operating room attire. As Dr Bill approached Beth, he simply walked right past, did not make eye contact with her, and went into the patient's room. Beth, left standing in the hall, experienced an awkward moment of exclusion and then took it upon herself to follow him into the room. When Dr. Bill entered the room, he failed to greet or look at the family members who stood around the patient's bed. Everyone moved away from the bed as Dr. Bill asked the patient what was wrong with his hand while moving back the sheet covering the patient's left hand. His assistant quietly stood by; Beth stood in the shadows against the wall.

Dr. Bill pulled out a Doppler and attempted to auscultate a radial pulse but was unable to do so. As he did this, he asked the patient about numbness in his hand. From against the wall, Beth quickly injected her assessment findings about significant numbness in the left hand, but neither she nor her words were acknowledged. At this point, Dr. Bill's assistant quietly mentioned that earlier in the morning an anesthesiologist had noticed that the patient's hand was blanched and numb. At this point Dr. Bill turned to the family and abruptly said, "He's got a clot in his hand; we need to take him back down and remove it." He said that "a nurse" (Beth was still in the room) would be in with a consent form and that the procedure would not take long. Dr. Bill turned to leave and as he did, one of the family members said, "We're so sorry to bother you. We know you are busy." Dr. Bill said nothing in response and walked out of the room and into the hall. His assistant soon followed. Beth stayed for a moment to assure the family that she would be right back. As Beth came out into the hall, Dr. Bill was well ahead. She followed him to the nurses' station and stood behind as he wrote orders in the patient's chart.

If I were to write a fictional account of what not to do when trying to build a team, I dare say I could not have written anything that comes close to this true story. Sadly, this scenario, in some form or another, occurs all too frequently on nursing units, where physicians, nurses, and patients interface on a regular basis.

Leaders' Role in Promoting Teamwork

What was the problem here, and where did Dr. Bill go wrong? First and foremost, I doubt whether Dr. Bill views himself as a team leader at all. He does not realize he is actively guiding a group that consists of some very important players on the unit: the patient, the patient's family, nursing staff, and ancillary staff.

Does Dr. Bill consider that his behavior, his demeanor, and the manner in which he interacts with others directly affects the accuracy, timeliness, and quality of communication that takes place, both current and subsequent? Does he understand that how he responds to feedback offered by his team is critical to whether he will receive feedback in the future regarding the condition of his patients? ◆

Dr. Bill does not understand any of this. The manner in which he responded on the phone to Beth's initial report of the patient's status was curt and dismissive. Rather than politely asking Beth for more details about her assessment, his response, "I just saw him," seemed defensive and laced with doubt. This sends Beth the message that her findings are not credible and reduces the chances that she will call again in a similar situation. Dr. Bill's abrupt declaration, "I'll be up," and then hanging up the phone lacks the basic respect and decorum that typifies professional conduct among team members. His response forces Beth to defend

---

◆ Sidebar 3.1
Leadership behavior and culture

Leaders play a critical role in creating, sustaining, and changing their organization's culture through their own behavior and through the programs and activities they support and praise or neglect and criticize.[1] However, the "primary embedding mechanisms" by which leaders' words and actions shape organizations culture are believed to be:

- What leaders pay attention to, measure, and control on a regular basis

- How leaders react to critical incidents

- Observed criteria by which leaders allocate scarce resources

- Deliberate role modeling, teaching, and coaching

- Observed criteria by which leaders allocate rewards and status

- Observed criteria by which leaders recruit, select, promote, retire, and ostracize organizational members[2]

Culture change has been found to be facilitated by demonstrated leader behavior and the team striving toward the production of a stable system of known values.[2, 4]

the very reason why she called in the first place, saying that she thought it was important enough for him to be informed.

The focus of this short, dysfunctional conversation now moves away from the patient and becomes a debate about whether a nurse should have provided a physician with feedback. How silly. Beth experiences the unsettling feeling that comes with having relevant patient information that must be acted upon, but is poorly received by the individual in charge.

When Dr. Bill comes to the unit and walks right by Beth without looking at her and enters the patient's room without her, he sends her a clear message that she is excluded from the team and not needed, which, of course, could not be further from the truth as far as the patient is concerned. When he fails to greet the patient and family and does not make eye contact, he sends a message of exclusion to them as well. Upon leaving the room, Dr. Bill completes his list of team-building transgressions by failing to stop and explain his findings to Beth and failing to give her positive feedback for a job well done. He also fails to assure the patient and family that they are not "bothering" him and that it is important and necessary for him to be informed if there are any concerns. Another telling part of this incident is the fact that Dr. Bill's nurse was previously aware that the patient's hand was blanched and numb, yet she had not shared these findings. It isn't too hard to figure out why.

Dr. Bill is probably a good surgeon and he surely desires good outcomes for his patients, but quite simply, he is not a good leader. He does nothing to foster collaboration and teamwork. In fact, some of his actions do great damage to the team's effectiveness.

This is the takeaway message here. Team effectiveness is about leadership, plain and simple. In this, or any case, the primary physician is the leader of the medical team. It is his or her responsibility to recognize the importance of demonstrating solid, well-planned leadership in all interactions with those delivering care to his or her patients at all levels of acuity. It is critical to know the individuals and job titles that make up the team, and it is just as important to recognize that the patient is a key part of that equation.

Effective leaders set a tone that fosters collaboration and open communication, and they work hard to maintain that atmosphere. They employ specific strategies and behaviors that facilitate information exchange and make it acceptable for anyone to speak up when something is not right. They encourage participation and are not threatened by questions or differing opinions. Remember, the initial research on airline disasters recognized failures in leadership as a direct cause; not poor technical prowess. Seeing oneself as a deity, beyond reproach and inquiry from subordinates, does not pass muster any more. Being rigidly task focused with little concern for human interaction will not work in high-risk endeavors.

We as nurses must demand solid leadership that incorporates team building behaviors from physicians as leaders of the medical team and from ourselves as leaders of the patient care team. (We will talk more about nurses as team leaders later on.) We can no longer accept or create excuses for poor behavior, citing personality quirks or eccentricities. On the contrary, these behaviors must be viewed as leadership failures in need of redirection and training. As we have seen with the airlines, the training is available, and cultures can change.

How the Airlines Accomplish Teamwork

At the airlines there is great emphasis on building and maintaining team effectiveness. Captains are taught to value their flight and cabin crews, and it is an accepted cultural paradigm that the best decisions are made when all members of the team are involved and provide accurate feedback. ◆ Captains are

◆ Sidebar 3.2
Structured communication

Studies have shown that leaders of teams with above-average performance ratings encourage team members to question their decisions and actions.[5] This is a distinct shift away from the belief that such behavior should be interpreted as a personal attack or insubordination. Instead, it is a shift to an understanding that such behavior is expected, and even demanded, from team members.[6]

In above-average teams, if a team member observes a suspected error in progress, the observer intervenes with a direct question or offer of information.[7] Actions of team members are challenged and safety concerns asserted in a manner that is not only appropriate, but expected.[8, 9] A key element of CRM is this type of purposefully structured, nonconfrontational communication that does not place blame on team members.[8] With repetition and reinforcement, the structured communication becomes habitual and the trust relationship between team members is strengthened.[10]

taught to know the resources at their disposal and to utilize them to the fullest whenever and wherever possible. Asking for help or considering another opinion is not weakness; it is sound leadership that puts operational safety before all else.

Let me illustrate. When I was a relatively new first officer at the airlines, I was riding what is called the jump seat, a small seat that folds down between the pilot and copilot seat in the cockpit. Occupying the jump seat is a privilege that pilots sometimes exercise to commute back and forth between their home city and the city in which they are based. In essence, it is a way to commute to home and work. On this particular night I was hitching a ride back to Memphis, TN, quietly observing the very experienced flight crew operate the aircraft and thinking about getting home.

As we approached the airport, the captain called for the landing gear to be lowered. As the first officer moved the landing gear handle to the down position, nothing happened. The first officer called out the problem and immediately referenced the aircraft's abnormal checklist as directed by the captain. He followed the instructions and recycled the handle by moving it up and then down again. Perhaps it was just some random quirk in the system, but still nothing. The crew informed air traffic control (ATC) of our problem and continued to run the abnormal checklist.

They followed every item to the letter, yet still there was no actuation; all three landing gear would not come down no matter what they did. The checklist now led the pilots to a section that was called emergency landing gear extension. This involved pulling a handle that blew out bolts and allowed the landing gear to free-fall into position. It was an irreversible action and was a one-shot deal. The captain called maintenance personnel on the ground to see whether they could shed some light on the situation. Their recommendation was to follow the checklist and to attempt the emergency extension.

As the crew started to review their actions and prepare for the emergency procedure, the captain paused and said out loud, "OK, what have we missed here? Is there anything we are forgetting or not seeing?" After a few seconds, he specifically turned to me and said, "Do you have any thoughts or suggestions?" ◆

I had seen this in the simulator before and had practiced this very scenario. I began to recall that during the simulator session, the instructor explained that it was possible to have a landing gear failure caused by a tripped circuit breaker; however, checking that circuit breaker was not an item listed on the abnormal checklist. In other words, nothing would tell the pilots to look there to solve the problem. I was not completely sure whether this was the issue here, but I responded to the captain by saying, "Have you checked all the circuit breakers? Perhaps that might make a difference." The captain turned to run his hand along the multiple lines of circuit breakers organized in rows just below his left shoulder. As he did so, he suddenly paused and said out loud, "Wait a minute." Moments later I heard the clunk of the landing gear as it began to cycle. Soon, the dimly lit cockpit was illuminated with three green lights. The gear was down and locked.

◆ Sidebar 3.3
Formed and fixed teams

One of the numerous ways to categorize teams is to describe them as fixed or formed:

- Formed teams: These are teams that come together for a relatively brief time to execute a specific task or project. They often are not together long enough to fully move through the familiar developmental stages of forming, storming, norming, and performing.[11] Airline crews and most surgical teams are examples of formed teams.

- Fixed teams: A nursing unit is an example of a fixed team. With the exception of float or agency personnel, most team members on nursing units expect future association with each other in the near term.

A study of airline crews compared fixed and formed crews and found that formed crews committed fewer minor errors but the number of major errors did not significantly differ between the two groups. The study's authors concluded that formed crews may have less complacency than fixed crews.[12] Still, when conditions dictate a need to juggle resources, dependency on others obviously increases. When there is a high probability of future association, as found in a fixed team, people are more likely to cooperate.[13, 14]

This story is CRM in action and illustrates superb leadership. The abnormal checklist was in the process of being redesigned to include the circuit breaker step; I just happened to have that knowledge from my recent training. Clearly, three heads were better than two in this case.

Here was a senior captain with years of experience, who had absolutely no reservations about asking a green and wet-behind-the-ears first officer riding his jump seat whether he had any suggestions about how to solve a perplexing situation in the cockpit. It was very impressive. I did not solve the problem; the captain did. He used all resources at his disposal and had no problems asking for suggestions; his call to maintenance personnel on the ground demonstrates this.

This example illustrates a phrase used to explain the operating mode of CRM, which is "use all available resources." Not some, or half, but "all" available resources. Good CRM dictates that people never let their ego get in the way of seeking input from the team. Just the fact that this captain stopped and asked the question "Are we missing something here?" suggests that he understands human fallibility. He knows that on any given day, under the right circumstances, important things can be missed regardless of experience or proficiency. He also understands that a countermeasure to this fact is to have other team members participating and giving feedback, offering suggestions, and pointing out discrepancies.

Part of the early mantra of CRM was "authority with participation." This correctly implies that authority is not weakened by team involvement, but enhanced. This one statement, if truly accepted in healthcare, would go a long way toward preventing harm to our patients. However, we know that on many fronts in healthcare, and certainly within the nursing experience (as with Beth and Dr. Bill), ego, rigid authority, and inappropriate behavior serve to mitigate and drive away resources. This is a cultural constant and places patients in danger. Here are some examples:

- A surgeon avoids actively conferring with an anesthesiologist and operating room team when deciding whether to continue a complicated case

Soaring to Success

- A nurse refuses to seek advice from other staff nurses when unsure about how to respond to unexplained changes in a patient's assessment

- An emergency room physician is slow to accept help after several failed attempts at intubation

- An intensivist dismisses suggestions from an ICU nurse regarding a patient's medication regimen because the physician feels that "a nurse should not tell him how to practice medicine"

- A staff nurse on a medical unit fails to accept input from a nurse's aide about a change in a patient's neurological assessment

- A chief nursing officer decides to add bed capacity to a step-down unit but never seeks input from the manager of the unit

In each of these examples, individuals are focusing heavily on themselves, not on the resources around them. In healthcare we focus heavily on competence, as we should. However, when we focus so much on individual competence and performance that we expect perfection, harshly judging the skill set of practitioners needing help in clinical situations, we do so at the patient's peril. At the airlines, pilots also focus heavily on skill set and individual competence. Yet pilots are looked upon favorably when they:

- Seek input from others before making decisions (time permitting)

- Seek help from others to manage human factor limitations (task overload)

Competence and seeking out help by using all resources are not mutually exclusive.

To conclude this point about resources, consider that at the airlines, the concept of team initially centered on those who occupied the cockpit. This later changed, expanding to include others such as flight attendants, flight dispatchers, mechanics, and ramp agents.

Anyone contributing to the flight is on the team and can freely share information that the pilot and copilot could use to make decisions about safety. The inclusion of this supporting cast of characters, along with a focus on the nuances of group interactions, led to the redefinition of the "C" in CRM from "cockpit" to "crew." The premise is that any member of the team is free to relay information to the captain in the interest of safety, and the focus is on behaviors that facilitate that process. Here is an example:

> *While the aircraft is at the gate with passengers actively boarding, a baggage handler notices a relatively large dent in the fuselage of the aircraft. He is not sure whether this is an abnormality that may cause a problem or not a big deal. To further complicate things, the flight has been delayed and everyone is anxious to get things moving.*

> *The baggage handler feels this information should be relayed to the captain. He radios to the lead ramp agent and the information is passed on to the captain, who promptly thanks the agent for the information. The captain then calls maintenance personnel to inspect the potential damage. Upon inspection it is revealed that the dent is quite severe and may have been caused by a collision with ground equipment or a service vehicle. Structural integrity of the fuselage is in question, and the flight is stopped at that point.*

Although this may be an inconvenience to passengers who were already experiencing delays, the sequence of events may have averted a disaster. The baggage handler at that moment was part of the "crew" and was empowered to bring this information to the captain. Imagine if clinical areas where physicians, nurses, and ancillary personnel function together consistently facilitated this kind of empowerment and teamwork. Think about the nursing assistant who sees a resident fail to sanitize his hands after leaving a patient's room. Does that nursing assistant feel free to present that information to the resident in the interest of safety? Does the culture support that? Will the physician view a challenge from a nursing assistant as an affront, or see her as a resource, preserving patient safety? Clearly, nosocomial infections can affect mortality on a much larger scale than a single airline disaster.

Some airlines require that pilots and flight attendants go through portions of their training together. This facilitates communication between the two groups and serves to clearly define the team. In the past, the cockpit door stood as a barrier between these two groups, but that is no longer the case. In January 2009, US Airways Captain Chesley "Sully" Sullenberger successfully ditched an Airbus 320 in the frigid Hudson River. Moments after the aircraft came to rest on the surface, with water rising in the cabin, both the cockpit and cabin crew executed a successful evacuation without a single fatality: truly remarkable. Captain Sullenberger later described in an interview that soon after making the announcement "Brace for impact," he heard the flight attendants chanting commands to the passengers over and over again, "Brace, brace, heads down, stay down." Sullenberger said that as he descended toward the water, he felt comforted by this; he knew immediately that the flight attendants were "on the same page." He knew that if he could land safely, they would get the passengers out of the aircraft; and they did. Captain Sullenberger was clearly in charge and making decisions, but he recognized that his expert skill alone would not avert disaster. He needed his team.

CRM delineates between dictatorial leadership styles that create apprehension and fear those that facilitate participation and inquiry. I like to think of it in simple terms; either you are a dictator or you are a facilitator, period.

As I encounter all kinds of leaders in healthcare—physicians, nurses, executives—I must admit that I quietly classify them through the prism of CRM and place them in one of the two categories. To emulate the facilitator, leaders in the cockpit learn specific behaviors, strategies, and techniques, which serve to empower team members in such a way that they are compelled to join in and speak up when they have concerns about operational safety. These strategies and behaviors can be learned and applied by all clinicians in a multitude of healthcare scenarios.

Conclusion

In the next chapter we will examine some of these strategies and behaviors. As we do, keep in mind that in many clinical situations the team may look different at times; and while the characters and venue may change, no version of a healthcare team is less critical to patient safety than another.

In a procedural-based area such as an operating room or cardiac catheterization lab, the team is physically together in one place; they are functioning together in a time-constrained environment that is high risk, potentially dynamic, and safety sensitive. In a sense, it almost feels like a cockpit, which is why CRM exports so well to these areas. In an ICU or medical-surgical nursing unit, the team—consisting of registered nurses, practical nurses, technicians, nursing assistants, physicians, and many others—are less often standing side by side, physically in the same space at the same time. Yet, the need for effective communication and teamwork in these areas remains high 24/7 and is equally, if not more, crucial in the effort to keep patients free from harm.

References

1. Sine, D.M., N. Northcutt, Effects of organizational leadership behavior on learning ethics: A study of professional paramedics. *Journal of Emergency Management.* 2009; 7(6): p. 61–70.

2. Schein, E.H. *Organizational Culture and Leadership.* 3rd ed. 2004, San Francisco: Jossey-Bass.

3. Martin J. *Organizational Culture: Mapping the Terraine.* 2002, Thousand Oaks, CA: Sage.

4. Sine, D.M., N. Northcutt, A qualitative analysis of the central values of professional paramedics. *American Journal of Disaster Medicine.* 2008, 3(6).

5. Helmreich, R.L., J.A. Wilhelm, S.E. Gregorich, et al., Preliminary results from the evaluation of cockpit resource management training: performance rating of flight crews. *Aviation, Space, and Environmental Medicine.* 1990, 61: p. 576–9.

6. Musson, D.M., R.L. Helmreich, Team training and resource management in health care: Current issues and future directions. *Harvard Health Policy Review.* 2004, 5(1): p. 25–35.

7. Risser, D.T., M.M. Rice, M.L. Salisbury, The potential for improved teamwork to reduce medical errors in the emergency department. *Annals of Emergency Medicine.* 1999, 34: p. 373–83.

8. Marshall, D.A., D.A. Manus, A team training program using human factors to enhance patient safety. *AORN Journal.* 2007, 86(6): p. 994–1011.

9. Pizzi, L., N.I. Goldfarb, D.B. Nash, Crew Resource Management and its Applications in Medicine. In *Making Health Care Safer: A Critical Analysis of Patient Safety Practices Agency for Healthcare Research and Quality.* 2001, U.S. Department of Health and Human Services.

10. Lewicki, R., B.B. Bunker, Developing and Maintaining Trust in Work Relationships. In Trust in Organizations: Frontiers of Theory and Reasearch, R. Kramer and T. Tyler, Editors. 1996, Thousand Oaks, CA: Sage.

11. Tuckman, B. Developmental sequence in small groups. *Psychological Bulletin.* 1965, 63: p. 384–99.

12. Barker, J.M., C.C. Clothier, J.R. Woody, et al. Crew resource management: A simulator study comparing fixed versus formed aircrews. *Aviation, Space, and Environmental Medicine.* 1996, 67: p. 3–7.

13. Webb, E.J. Trust and Crisis. In Kramer RM, Tyler TR, eds. Trust in Organizations. Thousand Oaks: Sage; 1996: p. 292.

14. Powell W. Trust Based Forms of Governance. In: Kramer RM, Tyler TR, eds. Trust in Organizations: Frontiers of Theory and Reasearch, R. Kramer and T. Tyler, Editors. 1996, Thousand Oaks, CA: Sage, p. 293.

CHAPTER 4

Get Connected and Set the Tone

LEARNING OBJECTIVES

After reading this chapter, the participant will be able to:

- List leadership behaviors that encourage open communication

- Identify how nurse leaders set the tone for a unit

In the previous chapter, we discussed the importance of utilizing available resources, a hallmark of crew resource management (CRM). If the resources at our disposal are manuals or computer databases, we need only type on a keyboard or open a page to make use of it. But teams are comprised of people, our patient's most valuable resource. To optimize these human resources, there are specific steps leaders must take to ensure the team is participating and communicating fully.

People Skills

In the 1990s, National Aeronautics and Space Administration (NASA) did a study of airline captain and flight crew behavior over the course of several days of simulated flights.[1] One of the dimensions measured was "expressivity," the term for crew members' acumen in interpersonal skills, including interpersonal warmth and concern. One of many findings was the fact that crews led by captains with higher expressive traits—better interpersonal skills—made fewer errors. This supports the premise that interpersonal skills are a must if you are to be an effective leader. Keep in mind that the primary objective of early-generation CRM was to focus on the "interpersonal" aspects of flight.[2]

Greeting and connecting

So, how do you strategically use interpersonal skills to build teamwork and open communication? You must be polite and courteous. You must greet and acknowledge members of your team when you see them at the start of a shift. You must make eye contact with people, offer a smile, talk to them, and engage them early on. Pleasantly offering a sincere "good morning" or "good afternoon" immediately lays a great foundation for effective communication and feedback. Laying this foundation takes some effort, but effective leaders do it well.

I remember being a first officer at the airlines and arriving at the aircraft knowing I would be flying with a captain I had never met or worked with before. When captains greeted me with a smile, shook my hand, introduced themselves, and involved me in conversation, I felt like a valued member of the team right away.

Imagine you are a nursing assistant and you arrive on a surgical unit to start your shift. The RN you are working with fails to greet you, does not say "good morning" or "Hi, how are you?" She doesn't smile, look at you, or talk to you. How would you feel? Chances are, you will turn inward, perhaps feel slighted or even angry. As you stand near your dour team leader wading through the uncomfortable silence, subtle barriers begin to form. This situation does not bode well for effective communication throughout the shift.

Similar situations occur in operating room (OR) settings where communication can be less than optimal as surgical teams begin making incisions on patients when not all members of the team have spoken to, or made eye contact with each other.[3] Again, good leaders know their team and will make efforts to greet and engage them early on.

Greeting and connecting is not a personality trait reserved for only the most outgoing or gregarious of us; this is a strategy consciously employed by good leaders to build effective teams.

Listening

It is also important to listen well. This means that when you, as a leader, solicit feedback from someone on the team, you must really listen when it is provided. If you are not sincere, and your actions and posture show a different intent, communication and teamwork are jeopardized. However, when simple steps are taken to listen actively, the probability of information exchange significantly increases.

Take the case of a physician, Gina, who rounds early in the morning on a medical step-down unit. As Gina sits at the nurse's station reviewing her patient's chart, she sees the night nurse, Jim, standing in the vicinity, finishing up some end-of-shift work at a computer station. Gina approaches Jim, greets him by saying good morning, and asks about his night. He smiles and responds in kind with pleasantries. She then asks him how Mr. Jones, her patient who was transferred from the ICU the day before, is doing and inquires about his night. Jim is a true professional who takes pride in his work and pays great attention to detail. He has provided excellent care to Mr. Jones and has assessed his status thoroughly at close intervals throughout the night. As Jim provides a brief summary of Mr. Jones' status, Gina looks at him as he talks, nodding her head frequently with an occasional "yes" or "OK" to demonstrate that she has received and understands the information. She does not read or start writing in a patient's chart while Jim is talking, she doesn't start slowly walking away as if there is something more important to attend to, nor does she interrupt him impatiently wanting specific answers to an open-ended question. **She simply faces him, maintains appropriate eye contact, and listens.** This tells Jim that what he is saying is important, while sending the message that he is a valued member of the team. It increases the likelihood that at some point in the future he will provide important, perhaps critical, information to this physician when not prompted or asked, which is always a team leader's desired objective. This strategy also increases the chance that subtle but important patient data may actually be heard by the leader and acted upon by the team, an outcome often missing in clinical communication. The physician in this case values teamwork and knows how to use interpersonal skills to create it.

A brief word about eye contact. Generally 5 to 10 seconds of eye contact is about right to let someone know that you are interested and engaged in what he or she is saying. On the other hand, if you look at someone directly for much longer than that, things can begin to feel somewhat uncomfortable.

Although the leader portrayed in the scenario above is a physician (the leader of the medical team), the same onus for building teams applies to RNs, who are the leaders of the patient care team on nursing units. Therefore, it is imperative that RNs—whose direct teams comprise RNs, licensed practical nurses (LPN), nursing assistants, and ancillary staff— possess and employ a basic proficiency in interpersonal communication. This lays the groundwork for cooperation and open communication within the group.

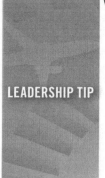

LEADERSHIP TIP

When forming and maintaining a team, effective leaders:

- Warmly greet members of the team at the start of the shift

- Smile

- Engage team members in conversation

- Set a polite and courteous tone

- Actively listen when receiving information

- Maintain a listening posture and appropriate eye contact

Setting the Tone

As a first officer sitting in the right seat of an airliner, I always knew that when the going got tough and I was unsure of the best decision, I could turn to my left and there would be someone sitting there to consult. When I upgraded to captain, I soon found that when I turned to my left, I saw my reflection in the side glass of the airplane. Airline captains understand the phrase "the captain sets the tone." This is something they learn early on, and it is absolutely true. It simply means that the manner in which the team functions, the template for doing work and making decisions, is set early on by the actions, words, and behaviors of the leader of the team and no one else.

If you are an RN who leads patient care teams on the unit, get out the mirror and take a look at your reflection. Just like the captain in the cockpit, the person staring back at you is responsible for setting the tone.

Previously, we discussed setting a polite and courteous tone. This means using good manners and demonstrating respect for all individuals on the team. While this seems simple enough, any seasoned nurse will acknowledge that nursing units can be hostile environments at times. The steady flow of patient and physician complaints, the rapid turnover of acutely ill patients, performance pressures from administration, coupled with the frustrations of inadequate staffing can push nurses to the brink. Given these realities, consistently setting a polite and courteous tone with the team becomes a real challenge requiring focused self-discipline, but, it is well worth the effort.

LEADERSHIP TIP	If operational pressures and negative forces cause a nurse leader to stop treating team members with respect, then all is lost and chaos reigns. Leaders must set the right tone, especially when the pressure is on.

How messages are sent

As a nurse leader on the unit, you set the tone through what you say and how you act, especially under pressure. Your words and behavior broadcast subtle messages to the team that they will file away as a reference for doing business on your watch. Let's look at the following example to illustrate the importance of setting the tone:

It's 2 p.m. on a 42-bed med-surg unit. The day has been extremely busy, with multiple admissions and discharges. Jennifer is the RN in charge of the unit in addition to handling a group of patients. Lea is an RN in her first year of practice. Lea has a patient who has developed a deep vein thrombosis (DVT) and is receiving a heparin infusion. A new bag of heparin needs to be hung, and the rate needs to be increased based on the last activated partial thromboplastin time (aPTT) value. Lea needs another nurse to go to the room with her and double-check the infusion, rate change calculation, and pump setting as required by protocol. Several nurses are at a late lunch, while others

are busy with patients and not available. Lea finds Jennifer and asks her to perform the
double-check. Jennifer responds by saying, "Go ahead and hang it. I trust you can follow
the protocol. I'll come down later when things settle down here."

Here Jennifer is setting a tone that says the following: Protocol and policy will be followed some of the time.

We must acknowledge the pressures on the unit and the fact that it's clearly not an optimal day: It's extremely busy, nurses are eating lunch at 2 p.m., and the charge nurse is responsible for managing operations while providing patient care; but, this cannot be used as rationale for dismissing protocol. Lea now internalizes that the template for doing work, at least with Jennifer as charge nurse, is somewhat permissive and open to interpretation when it comes to standards. You can picture Lea, perhaps a few months later, saying to herself, "I'll just go ahead and hang it. I can follow the protocol. I'll have someone check it later when things aren't so busy."

A more preferable scenario is one in which Jennifer not only stops what she is doing to double-check the infusion with Lea, but uses the situation as an opportunity to verbally reinforce the importance of adhering to standard operating procedures.

All nurses are leaders

If an RN constantly bad-mouths the nurse manager, criticizes administration, complains about staffing and the demanding nature of certain patients, then the LPNs and nursing assistants who follow her lead are likely to assume the same posture when providing care.

Setting the tone is a critical leadership behavior. When this behavior is executed improperly, or not at all, patients are exposed to unnecessary hazards.

The Grid

The tone that leaders set is the embodiment of their leadership style. To illustrate this point, some CRM programs focus on the managerial grid proposed by Blake and Mouton back in the 1960s (See Figure 4.1).[4]

FIGURE
4.1

Leadership Grid

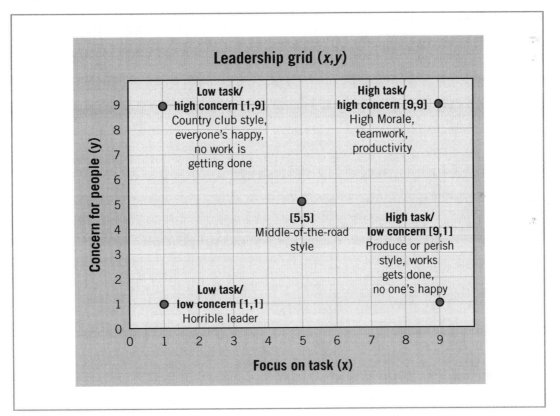

Put simply, this provides a frame of reference for leaders to plot their leadership style. The grid rates one's focus on task (*x* axis) on a scale of 1 through 9, with 9 being the highest. It also rates concern for people (*y* axis) on this same 1 through 9 scale. Here are the various types of leaders:

- High task/low concern: These leaders focus only on the tasks to be completed (produce or perish style)

- Low task/high concern: These leaders show concern only for people and their feelings (country club style)

- Low task/low concern: These leaders show little concern for task or people (horrible leader)

- High task/high concern: These leaders have high concern for both people and task (high morale, teamwork, and productivity)

- Neither high nor low task/concern: These leaders settle for mediocrity and are termed middle of the road, willingly sacrificing some team morale and productivity to simply carry on

The NASA research mentioned earlier demonstrates that captains who focus only on performance with little concern for interpersonal elements (high task/ low concern; expressed as a 9, 1 on the grid orientation), got poorer performance from their crew when compared to captains with both a high concern for people as well as task performance.

This likely makes sense to you and supports the idea that to have effective team performance, leaders must balance these two concerns. Let's look at the leadership grid more closely and apply it to the nursing unit.

Nurses and the leadership grid

Imagine you are an RN in charge of seven patients on the day shift. You walk into one of your patient's rooms to administer medications and see that the patient's face appears grayish–blue in color. You immediately determine that the patient is not breathing so you call for help and start CPR. As you perform compressions on the patient's chest, other staff members enter the room. You clearly and with authority make eye contact with specific individuals, nod your head forward, and say the following:

"Don, get the crash cart immediately. Plug it in and place leads on the patient to start cardiac monitoring. Susan, I want you to start an IV. Terry, I want you to check with the unit clerk to be sure that a code has been called and then continue to monitor the rest of the floor. Tom, I want you to get the O$_2$ and suction set up. Let's go! Let's move!"

Where would you plot this nurse team leader on the grid? If you said high task/low concern I would agree (see Figure 4.2). Is this appropriate? If your response is that in this circumstance, it is appropriate for the nurse team leader to behave in this manner, I would also agree. The situation is critical, it dictates that specific tasks be completed promptly. Can you imagine the nurse in this situation saying, "Don, would you mind getting the crash cart for me? Are you OK with that?" That would be ludicrous. Here, high task/low concern leadership is required and the nurse operationalizes that by staying task focused. ◆

Now consider a different scenario. You are the evening shift charge nurse responsible for the management of patient care on a 37-bed surgical unit. One of the RNs working with you is consistently professional and thorough when completing her work. You have counted on her many times in the past to safely manage the multiple admissions and postoperative arrivals that characterize the evening shift. Today, however, things are different. She appears flustered and it is becoming clear to you that she is falling behind in the completion of required tasks. You are concerned about the safety of her

> ◆ **Sidebar 4.1**
> ## Leaders and crisis decisions
>
> How do people make decisions in a crisis? Classic models for decision making follow a process in which several options are identified, the options are weighed and ranked based on criteria, and after a deliberative process the option with the highest score is selected.[5–7]
>
> In a crisis situation, however, there is rarely time or sufficient information for the classic decision model to work. Experienced leaders see a situation, even one that is nonroutine, as an example of a familiar prototype and see a course of action right away. This approach to problem solving, called recognition-primed decision making, allows decision makers to pursue a workable solution to a crisis immediately without having to weigh the advantages and disadvantages of a set of options. The emphasis is on being poised to act, rather than being paralyzed as all the evaluations are completed.[8]

patients. In this situation, you elect to take the nurse aside, away from others, and ask her, in a supportive manner, about the situation. You inquire whether there is anything wrong or whether something is bothering her. You soon find out that she has experienced a death in the family and is not coping well. You determine that she cannot continue and decide to assume the care of her patients. Here, high task/low concern leadership is inappropriate. You don't berate this nurse or pressure her to work harder and faster. You focus on the person and correctly demonstrate low task/high concern leadership (see Figure 4.2).

FIGURE
4.2

Leadership Grid 2

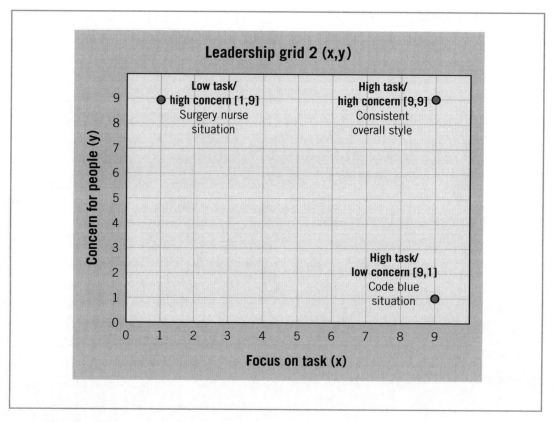

The overriding point is that for each situation you encounter as a leader, there is an optimal place to reside on the grid regarding leadership focus and tone. Each leader must decide where that is.

Team effectiveness is degraded when we fail to correctly match situation with tone. Just as airline captains are urged to evaluate their planned response to each situation using the grid, nurses can do the same.

In addition to being a situational assessment of leadership, you can use the grid to plot one's overall style of leadership. As a nurse leader, if your day-to-day style offers a good balance of focus on task and concern for people, then your chances of being effective are enhanced and your team will understand when your leadership tone changes to meet situational variability. Focusing only on feelings and having multiple group hugs will not garner respect. Screaming and yelling constantly about performance measures and tasks may get results for a while, but not in the long run. On the other hand, consistently gravitating through word and action to the upper right part of the leadership grid offers the best chance for setting the best tone for teamwork and safety.

A Point about the NASA Study and Healthcare

The NASA study discussed earlier supports the value of a captain who sets a tone that is explicit about the reality that there are tasks to complete, but also employs behaviors that send a clear message to team members that their input is valued, desired, and critical to success.

It is interesting to note that over time, the crews that experienced a leader with a high task/low concern grid style (task focused only, with little concern for interpersonal relationships) started out with subpar performance but rebounded to an acceptable level over time—not as good as the team led by the high task/high concern captain, but an acceptable adaptation nonetheless. This is very interesting when we move into healthcare. Nurses must endure physicians and fellow nurses who set inappropriate leadership tones coupled with a high task/low concern style on a routine basis. Just think about the surgeon who barks orders consistently, refuses to hear contrary opinions, and has little concern for the thoughts and feelings of others. If this behavior goes unchecked, whether in the OR or out on the nursing units, nurses are forced to adapt and employ workarounds to maintain some level of performance and safety for their patients. In this regard, performance rebounds to an acceptable level, but not an optimal one.

In healthcare, we accept poor leadership styles from both physicians and nurses. We accept practitioners who demonstrate little concern for people. We accept clinical leaders who set an awful tone, and like the airline pilots in the NASA research, force the team to adapt. A better solution is a move toward creating leaders who effectively balance both task orientation and concern for people both in medicine and nursing. In 2009, The Joint Commission introduced Leadership Standards that require a focus on interpersonal skills and professionalism in medical staff core competencies, along with zero tolerance for poor behavior. Addressing this issue directly in the standards is long overdue, but clearly a step in the right direction. Joint CRM training for nursing and medical students is a much better solution to create better healthcare leaders.

References

1. Chidester, T., et al. Personality Factors in *Flight Operations: Volume I: Leader Characteristics and Crew Performance in a Full-Mission Air Transport Simulation,* 1990, Moffet Field, CA. NASA Technical Memorandum 102259, NASA-Ames Research Center.

2. Helmreich, R.L. Culture and error in space: Implications from analog environments. *Aviation, Space, & Environmental Medicine,* 2000. 71(9, Section 2 Suppl): p. A133–A139.

3. Marshall, D., and D. Manus, A team training program using human factors to enhance patient safety. *AORN Journal,* 2007. 86(6): p. 994–1011.

4. Helmreich, R., and H. Foushee, Why crew resource mangement? Empirical and theoretical bases of human factors training in aviation, in *Cockpit Resource Management*, E. L. Wiener, Editor. 1993, San Diego, CA: Elsevier, p. 3–41.

5. Head, G., and S. Horn, *Essentials of Risk Management,* Vol. 1. 1997, Malvern, PA: Insurance Institute of America.

6. Janis, I.L., and L. Mann, *Decision Making: A Psychological Analysis of Conflict, Choice, and Commitment.* 1977, New York: Free Press.

7. Soelberg, P.O., Unprogrammed decision making. *Industrial Management Review,* 1967. 8: p. 19–29.

8. Klein, G., *Sources of Power: How People Make Decisions.* Cambridge, MA: MIT Press.

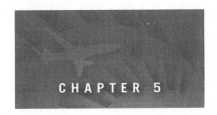

CHAPTER 5

Improve Team Cohesiveness With Briefings

LEARNING OBJECTIVES

After reading this chapter, the participant will be able to:

- Explain the principles of leadership briefings

- Describe how nursing unit briefings improve teamwork

In Chapter 4, we discussed key crew resource management (CRM) strategies such as using interpersonal skills and setting the tone. Now let's build on that and examine how the use of briefings provide opportunities for nurse team leaders to set the appropriate tone and create a foundation for effective team communication.

When a team comes together—whether at the start of a flight or the start of a shift—it should begin with a briefing. Whether the teams consists of one person, five, or more, conducting a briefing is an excellent leadership and team-building strategy. Briefings conducted early on with the entire team are critical to team effectiveness. Briefings set expectations, clarify roles and responsibilities, and, when conducted properly, set the tone that we described in Chapter 4: task focused, but also relaxed and people focused so others feel comfortable speaking up when necessary.

An indicator of the effectiveness of an airline crew is heavily based on what captains do in the first few minutes after the team comes together.[1] At the airlines, it is common for captains to brief the copilot and the flight attendants. This can be done separately, but is often done together. The captain does this right away, shortly after the team meets on the aircraft for the first time. Any or all of the following items will be covered:

- Departure

- En route and destination weather

- Expected time aloft

- Expected turbulence

- Cockpit security

- Review of communication and emergency procedures

- Any crew member's questions or concerns

Airlines can employ thousands of pilots, and crews frequently arrive at an aircraft prior to flight to discover at least some members of the team have never met or seen each other before. When there is no prior rapport or relationship with crew members, it is vital for captains to promptly begin the team-building process. First, they extend greetings and introductions to the crew, which is followed by a team briefing. This is done every day, over and over again in cockpits throughout the world, and is an excellent strategy to increase the chances that the crew will successfully identify and manage potential threats to safety.

In healthcare, the use of briefings is a key component of CRM-based initiatives being exported to the operating room (OR). Surgeons are taught to greet their team and then conduct a briefing about the case with all members present: circulating nurses, technicians, and anesthesia providers. In the Veteran's Administration, the Medical Team Training program teaches OR teams to develop and use a preoperative briefing to enhance teamwork and communication. In 2009, the World Health Organization published a study that demonstrated significant reductions in perioperative morbidity and mortality with the use of a checklist before surgery, much like pilots use in the cockpit.[2, 3] The initial result of the study showed the rate of surgical complications fells by 36% and deaths fell by 47% with use of the checklist. A key component on that checklist is team introductions and a briefing of anticipated events by the surgeon prior to incision. Over the past decade, proprietary companies throughout the country have taught CRM-based concepts to OR and other procedural-based healthcare teams, again with a major component of these programs concentrating on the development and use of team briefings.

Briefings on the Nursing Unit

CRM-based briefings can and should be used outside the OR wherever healthcare professionals work together to deliver and manage patient care. This is especially true on medical–surgical nursing units where activity occurs at a fever pitch, patient acuity is high, and the need for effective communication remains constant 24/7. ◆

When implemented appropriately, briefings can have a profound effect on the quality of communication and collaboration within healthcare teams; however, I have also seen the briefing concept misinterpreted and implemented

◆ Sidebar 5.1

Communicating key intent with briefings

The different professional cultures present in a multi-disciplinary team and unique perspective of the individual team members can produce a sort of "line friction" in channels of communication during task execution. Divergent perceptions and translations errors will make some amount of miscommunication between team members all but inevitable.[4–6] In addition, a complex operating environment, such as a nursing unit invariably contains multiple goals that can all be competing for attention simultaniously.[7]

Therefore, team briefings are particularly relevant to healthcare. These short synopses of intended actions by the individual in charge improve teamwork, communication, decision-making, and situational awareness.[8] Briefings were a specific recommendation of the Institute of Medicine's 2000 report *To Err is Human: Building a Safer Healthcare System*.[9] Briefings successfully applied in the OR setting have been shown to improve communication between surgeons and OR teams.[10–13] improperly in practice. This ultimately yields communication that falls short of what is intended.

Let's look at some key points about briefings and discuss application to the nursing environment. An effective briefing should be:

- **Short:** Briefings are designed to be succinct. This is relative, of course. For example, a briefing by a nurse to a nursing assistant at the start of a shift, or a surgeon prior to making an incision, may be three to five minutes in length. A briefing by a nurse to a patient before starting an IV or a physician to a nurse in a cardiac step down area may be shorter. The exact time required to brief is not important. However, if you find yourself talking on and on, and five minutes becomes 15, then the briefing threshold has been crossed. The point is, keep it short.

- **Informative:** Briefings should not be idle chat. They have a specific purpose, which is to convey important information. When briefing the team, you must have a clear idea of the salient and necessary points the team must know. Insignificant or superfluous information can create confusion and de-emphasize previously stated goals for the task at hand.

- **Structured:** Briefings are not free verse and open-ended, with several people talking all at once about their point of interest. On the contrary, briefings are led by one person, usually the individual in charge, and follow a predetermined format. This makes sense. If there is a lot of information to be delivered in a short period of time, using a template or outline ensures that the briefer stays on track and the team remains focused. The best method for providing structure to a briefing is the use of a briefing checklist. Although it is possible to remember the checklist via the use of an acronym, it is best to have it written down and carried for reference. When I was an airline captain, I used a pocket-sized laminated checklist when conducting the preflight briefing with the flight attendants and first officer. This worked well because it enabled me to stay organized and consistent, especially when I was feeling rushed or pressured between flights.

RN briefings

When I was a nurse manager of a medical–surgical unit, we piloted just such a briefing checklist to be used by the RNs to brief the nursing assistants. Traditionally, these two groups have not always communicated optimally. In many institutions, nursing assistants/ aides do not attend the change-of-shift report and often receive patient information as an afterthought. On our unit, we implemented the use of a laminated briefing card with key patient care items that the nurses used to brief the aide they would be working with on their shift.

The briefing card was in a checklist format and was pocket-sized; many nurses affixed them to their ID badges. The expectation was that after RNs received change of shift report, they would locate the nursing assistant and conduct the briefing using the card. The RNs would simply discuss each patient in their group relative to the items on the checklist. This was NOT report; it was a briefing covering only specific information. To create the briefing checklist, we simply asked RNs what they wanted the nursing aides to know and we asked nursing aides what they wanted the RNs to tell them. We asked both groups to name the items that often got overlooked or not communicated when providing care. (See Figure 5.1 for a template of a briefing checklist.)

How well did this work? The use of this checklist was part of a larger pilot study, and one of several interventions; therefore, it is difficult to relate any specific metric to the checklist alone. I remain convinced, however, that the reaction of the RN staff was the most interesting finding. It was, in essence, the clash of two professional cultures when it came to the use of a formalized briefing and checklist: aviation and nursing. Some of the nurses accepted the checklist and found it helpful, while others completely ignored it. Still others used it intermittently and admitted feeling silly referencing a checklist for something they always did from memory. There were two nurses that specifically stand out in my mind.

Each expressed identical sentiment: "Do I have to use the checklist every time?" "I've been a nurse for 20 years; I know what I want to tell them [the nursing assistants]." "It seems ridiculous to just keep looking at the checklist over and over."

FIGURE
5.1

RN to Nursing Assistant Briefing Checklist

This is a template of a briefing card with key patient care items that nurses can use to brief nursing assistants with whom they will be working.

RN to Nursing Assistant Briefing Checklist

❏ Safety risks

    ❏ Bed alarm

    ❏ Falls

    ❏ Restraints

❏ Priority turns

❏ Specimens

❏ NPO

❏ Fluid restrictions

❏ Feeding assistance

❏ Daily weights

❏ Vital sign issues

My response: "What if you were traveling on an airplane to go on vacation. As you taxi out to the runway, anticipating the excitement that lies ahead, you hear the captain's voice over the intercom. 'Well folks welcome on board, this is the captain. We hope you have a good flight with us today. I want you to know that the copilot and I have been flying for a combined 45 years and we feel that we have the routine procedures required to fly this airplane memorized. Therefore, on today's flight we're gonna try something new. We will not be using any checklists, briefings, or formal methods of communication.' Would you sit back and relax as the pilot suggests? You might sit back, but I doubt you would relax!"

I then continued with a more germane question: "In your many years of nursing have you ever been involved in a situation where a patient had a procedure or diagnostic test postponed because they received a food tray when their status was NPO?" Their answer was predictable. "Well, yeah, but …" I then made the point to them that maybe our communication as nurses isn't always as effective as we might think. The purpose of the briefing checklist is to formalize communication to ensure that nothing is missed. ◆

Briefing Checklists

Notice that one of the items on the briefing checklist is "specimens." If you have ever

---

◆ Sidebar 5.2
Skipping the checklist

Even when checklists are used, it is possible that steps within the checklist—or even whole checklists—may inadvertently be skipped. Such omissions are most often the result of a disruption of normal duties or an effort to save time by taking shortcuts. However, even the continual repetition of a standardized process for checklist use can breed complacency.[14]

The following have also been identified as some of the reasons for partial or complete omission of a checklist:

- Changes in normal timing such as a delay

- Distractions

- Task saturation

- Management of priorities

- Reduced attention

- Inadequate task coordination and cross-check between team members

- Over-reliance on memory

- Less-than-optimum checklist content

- Inadequate emphasis on checklist use during training[15]

---

practiced nursing on multibed medical–surgical unit, you know that opportunities for specimen collection (stool, urine, sputum, 24-hour urine) are often missed because someone on the team was not aware that a collection for laboratory analysis had been ordered. This is significant when a debilitated patient 12 hours into a 24-hour urine collection must start all over again because the nursing assistant threw a specimen away, unaware that collection was in progress. The increased lengths of stay for these patients waste resources and unnecessarily expose them to hospital-acquired threats. These, and all the other acts of commission and omission, have a much better chance of being avoided with the use of a structured briefing by nursing staff.

And yes, most pilots do know their routine checklists by memory, the product of doing them over and over again. But they understand that checklists used along with standardized communication ensure that key steps of a safety critical process are not omitted.

Briefing checklists back up the human memory, which has limited capacity, especially when stressors are introduced.

"Do I have to use the checklist?"

No pilot would ever say such a thing out loud. Not only would it be absurd, it would be professional suicide. Yet, as we discussed, many nurses responded to the briefing checklists by saying just such a thing, rationalizing that their years in practice and their memories alone were far better than formal briefings and check-lists. It should give us all reason to pause when we realize that what would be considered ridiculous in the aviation culture—one that enjoys a high degree of operational safety—is a day-to-day reality in our own. Casual, informal communication from memory has no place when lives are at stake. ◆

> ◆ Sidebar 5.3
> ## Checklists: Memory and habit
>
> We commonly call unintended failures of execution slips, lapses, trips, or fumbles. Slips relate to observable actions and are commonly associated with attentional or perceptional failures. Lapses are internal events and generally involve failures of memory.[16]
>
> The use of checklists should become an embedded pattern or habit to avoid slips and lapses. The habitual use of a checklist is different from memorizing the steps contained in a checklist. Memory-guided checklist use (executing the steps in a checklist from memory) is not reliable and may devolve into a motor association response of holding or touching a checklist while going through memorized steps, often with steps missing or out of order.[14]

Opportunity to ask questions

As mentioned previously, briefings must be structured, conducted, and directed by the individual in charge. This means that for the most part one person talks and others listen. If there are constant interruptions or tangential issues enter the process, time for ensuring precise communication about the task at hand is lost. However, this cannot be taken to the extreme or out of context. A briefing is not a lecture during which those in attendance are expected to be seen, not heard. Effective briefings always allow for questions and clarifications from the team.

When giving a briefing, solicit feedback and check for understanding throughout. Ask the team, "Does anybody have any questions or concerns about what we've just discussed?" Or, "Is there anything anyone can think of that we haven't covered?" When feedback is requested in this manner, it is important to be sincere; the team needs to sense that you really want them to bring things forward. If you really don't want to hear from the team and you are simply saying words in a perfunctory fashion, the team will know and take mental notes. The key is to be structured, professional, and focused while clearly eliciting feedback.

Mental Model

The objective of any briefing is to establish a shared mental model. We hear the term quite a bit, but what does it mean? At face value it sounds like it means that all members of the team share common ideas about a situation or task. While this is true, a closer examination of the term is required.

Let's first start by discussing how a mental model affects our thought process and actions. Think about a nurse, Tom, caring for a patient with congestive heart failure (CHF). Tom has a mental image of the patient's cardiovascular and respiratory system; he visualizes the anatomy and understands the physiology. This is analogous to a pilot's mental image and understanding of a hydraulic or electrical system on an aircraft. Tom envisions the effect of pathology on the system. In his mind, he visualizes the weakened left ventricle struggling to eject oxygenated blood to body tissues, causing pressure to build in the heart. Tom understands that increased venous pressure and backflow causes fluid to leak out into tissues, which results in edema. He has an image of increasing pulmonary capillary pressure as fluid collects in the interstitial spaces of the pulmonary vasculature.

This is the nurse's mental model, or schematic, of the body system, which he then uses to manage this clinical problem. The mental model is burned in his long-term memory and guides his assessments and implementations. If the patient with CHF suddenly has difficulty, the nurse draws subconsciously on that mental model and responds by performing actions that are appropriate for the situation, such as repositioning the patient for comfort, ensuring the delivery of oxygen, checking vital signs, auscultating lung fields, assessing for edema, evaluating the medication regimen for appropriate therapy (diuretics, ACE inhibitors, and digoxin), reviewing electrolyte values, checking for arrhythmias, and notifying the physician whether further assessment or a change in medical orders is required.

Put simply, having a mental model allows us to know what the system looks like normally, what it looks like in an abnormal condition, and it guides us in knowing how to respond. It tells us what to examine and what to look for. It lets us know what to expect and aids us in understanding why something may be happening. A mental model provides a knowledge foundation that we apply to clinical situations in order to problem solve and make decisions. Without it, we are lost. ◆

Although mental models exist for a specific system in the body or in a jet aircraft, they can also be applied broadly to a multitude of clinical situations and processes. For example, early on, nurses

> ◆ Sidebar 5.4
> ## Competencies of team members
>
> Metaphors for teams abound. Klein, Zsambok, and Thordsen have proposed that teams mature along dimensions similar to those used to describe child development: competencies, identity, cognitive skills, and metacognition (reflective thinking about how the team learns, performs, and interacts). Competencies, or the abilities of team members to perform basic tasks, can greatly influence team performance. Team member mastery of the basics must be assured through recurrent training and assessment. Any evaluation of a team's ability to collaborate, exchange information, and form a shared mental model must also consider the individual team member's level of skill, particularly if the team's members keep changing.[17, 18]

learn the process used to admit a patient to an inpatient unit in the hospital. It has specific steps and handoffs, which have been reinforced over time by observation and repetition. It becomes their mental model for admission. This is why nurses swiftly intervene when an unstable patient just shows up on their unit without notification or medical orders (which does occasionally happen). Their mental model allows them to know what should have occurred along the way and that key points in the admission process were not followed. The nurse then backtracks through the process to procure the appropriate level of care for the patient.

Shared Mental Model

In a team situation, a briefing ensures that the mental model to be used is shared by all. A shared mental model guides the actions and awareness of not just one individual but the entire team. It gets team members on the same page, generates mutual understanding, and provides a working blueprint for getting the job done. Establishing the shared mental model requires that

specific items are covered in the briefing. The overall goal(s) of the team needs to be stated. This provides a big picture; it cuts through all the noise and places the most important objectives prominently in the minds of those on the team. This is important because, when team members are in a position where they must make a decision about what to do or how to respond in a clinical situation, they can draw from the mental model and default to actions that are most aligned with the stated goals. ◆

◆ Sidebar 5.5
Mental models and task anticipation

Individuals use mental models to describe, explain, and predict their surroundings. Formed mental models are made up of information in context and the relationships between the information elements.

When team members interact, their mental models converge.[19, 20] A team's shared knowledge structure enable them to form accurate explanations and expectations for the task, coordinate their actions with other team members, and adapt their behavior to the demands of the task.[20] The shared mental model of the task and the roles other team members will play allows an individual member of the team to anticipate what others are and will be doing. This allows each team member to keep mentally (and sometimes physically) ahead of a dynamic situation and not fall prey to information overload.[17]

Outlining big picture goals in the briefing allows for team members to make decisions independently when required and refocus others when actions stray from stated objectives. Let's briefly return to the OR setting to provide a simple example. A surgeon is performing a procedure that requires the use of a laser in a patient's airway where oxygen flow creates a fire risk. He briefs the OR team and clearly states that a big goal for the procedure is to avoid an intra-airway fire. Oxygen concentrations must be reduced to room air when ignition sources are present. At some point during the procedure, the surgeon is about to use the laser but becomes so immersed in the task at hand that he fails to call for a reduction in oxygen concentrations. The anesthesiologist, is also sidetracked administering medication to the patient and fails to promptly reduce oxygen flow. The circulating nurse remembers the goal that was emphasized in the briefing (not having an intra-airway fire) and immediately calls for the team to stop and for the anesthesiologist to reduce oxygen concentrations. The surgeon responds by saying, "Oh yes, thanks," and the anesthesiologist willingly complies. No one argues or pushes back because a "nurse is telling him what to do." The team simply acts because the mental model is shared.

How to conduct briefings

As an RN briefing your patient care team on the unit, ask yourself, "What are the main goals for this shift?" and communicate that in the briefing. The goal may simply be to not become complacent because the census is down. It could be to resist the temptation to take shortcuts because the census is up and you are short-staffed. Also, ask yourself whether there are big-picture goals for particular patients that need to be included in the briefing. Maybe it is ensuring that a frail and timid patient ambulates postoperatively. Maybe it is controlling intractable pain. Perhaps it is protecting a neutropenic patient from infection, or helping someone deal with the shock of a recent cancer diagnosis. If team members have big-picture information, they can choose actions that are both safe and appropriate when managing certain clinical situations.

It is also important to clearly define the rules for engagement, or the template that will be used by all team members to guide their behavior. At the airlines, a cockpit briefing always includes a variation of this simple statement: "We will follow standard operating procedures at all times." This short sentence is categorical; it leaves nothing to the imagination and takes the guesswork out of the process. This is critical when attempting to establish a shared mental model. During the flight, if the first officer is tempted to operate the aircraft in a nonstandard manner, he or she will recall the behavioral expectations set by the captain in the briefing and refrain from doing so. If there is a requirement to operate the aircraft in a manner inconsistent with standards (which can happen occasionally), this will be briefed and agreed upon first. Standard operating procedures in an aircraft are analogous to the policies and procedures found in healthcare. On any healthcare team, a briefing must include statements which make it clear that policies will be followed at all times. Consider this case in point. Five East is a medical–surgical unit that has instituted a safety briefing for all staff prior to change-of-shift report. The briefing is led by the charge nurse and reviews safety items and concerns on the unit for the upcoming shift. One of the items covered in the briefing is whether there are high-risk medications being infused on the unit. The patient's names, room number, and drug infusing are highlighted in the briefing. The charge nurse says the following two sentences to the team:

> *"To everyone, we must follow all clinical policies and procedures as we do our work today, no shortcuts. This especially means that all high-risk medications must be double-checked by two nurses before infusion rates are changed or initiated."*

This makes it clear to the entire team that whatever they do, whatever their job title, whether they are alone or in the presence of other team members, they are expected to do things by the book. Nurses well understand that there are times when attempting to do things by the book actually invites pejorative comments from peers. In a culture that is perpetually rushed, "by the bookers" can be seen as creating unnecessary delays or labeled as having poor time management skills. We must move away from this mind-set in nursing. An effective briefing delivered by a skilled nurse leader emulates the airline captain who says, "We will follow standard operating procedures at all times." This raises the standard in nursing and serves to reduce the risk of patient harm.

It is also important that the briefing discusses the roles and expectations of those on the team. This provides clarity when the team is facing situations that require prompt action. I remember my days in the cockpit and think of specific examples in which roles were clarified in a short briefing. As I mentioned previously, airline captains provide a general briefing to the first officer in the cockpit before flight deck duties commence, most often occurring when the crew first comes together to fly a trip. One of the items covered in this briefing is what to do in the case of an emergency and subsequent evacuation. Standard operating procedures call for the captain to fly the aircraft in the event of an emergency, and for the first officer to leave the cockpit and assist with an evacuation of the cabin should that be necessary. This is covered by the captain in the briefing and sounds something like this:

> *"If we lose an engine on takeoff, fly the aircraft according to standard operating procedures. Once stabilized, I will take control of the aircraft, and you will run the appropriate checklist. In the event of an evacuation, once we come to a stop, we will evacuate on my command. You will assist the evacuation, and I will complete the evacuation checklist."*

This is very important in developing a shared mental model. It clearly reviews and clarifies who is going to do what in the event of an emergency. Team members already know what is expected of them, and the briefing is not a time for teaching and learning to take place with regard to basic job responsibilities. It is, however, a time to emphasize the big picture when it comes to defining roles on the team, a time to bring the team back to the basics. Doing this allows key roles to be easily recalled in the heat of battle. This is important because the practical realities of everyday operation tend to put distance between operators and standard policies and procedures. ◆

◆ Sidebar 5.6
A dynamic mental model

Team cognition can be described as simply the ability of the team to reach a shared understanding of their situation. Is there agreement regarding goals and intents? What assumptions, such as who will fly the aircraft or the role of the primary responder, are guiding their actions? The mental model, however, is not static and must necessarily evolve as the situation changes. During response to dynamic emergency situations, many unanticipated events may occur that necessitate the rapid reformation of the mental model in response to the new conditions. The strength of the team is in its ability to respond to new and unexpected conditions and to draw upon the experience of the team members to generate performance that is beyond the capabilities of any individual member.[17, 21]

Roles during a briefing

Let's move to nursing and examine an area where roles can be clarified in a briefing to reinforce a shared mental model. Nurses who have worked in a medical–surgical setting are familiar with the confusion that can occur in a code blue situation on the unit, where a patient requires CPR and subsequent advanced cardiac life support (ACLS). Nurses on these units have multiple patients who can be extremely ill; their task load is high, and their ability to monitor patients closely is often compromised. Many times, nurses will simply find a patient unresponsive and have to literally call for help and begin CPR. The patient's room can become flooded with people as more and more personnel throughout the hospital arrive. What can be crucial to patient outcome, however, is what occurs in those first few minutes when nurses on the unit discover the patient. There are key steps that need to occur or be verified so that when the ACLS team arrives, resuscitation can promptly begin. This requires a clarification of roles. A perfect opportunity to do this is in the unit safety briefing during which safety items are reviewed by the charge nurse prior to each shift with all staff present. Here the charge nurse achieves a shared mental model by covering role expectations in a code blue situation:

> *"If we have a code blue today, everyone remember their primary roles. The first responder who finds the patient will initiate a call for help and immediately begin CPR. The first responder will direct others as they enter the room to achieve the following: obtain the crash cart, ventilate the patient with an ambu bag, establish intravenous access, hook up oxygen, place combo pads on the patient, and hook up suction (reference your code blue first-responder checklist). When the patient's primary nurse arrives, he or she remains in the room to verify that these actions are taking place and is available to provide pertinent medical history to the ACLS team. One nursing assistant and one licensed nurse will remain on the unit to meet the needs of other patients. The unit secretary will remain at the front desk area and verify that the ACLS team has been called and is en route. One nursing assistant will be available to procure supplies and meet other requests.*

You may be thinking this is unrealistic, or perhaps overkill. I urge you to think again. I assert that code blue ACLS situations on medical surgical units would have better outcomes with the use of such a briefing. Emergency situations rarely unfold in a neat and orderly fashion with every team member performing on cue. Physiologic responses may cause us to experience momentary panic or fear. These responses must be quelled, and we must quickly focus our attention to perform the task at hand. This is precisely why a briefing that establishes a shared mental model by highlighting roles is so valuable. Team members can recall and default to these roles with little thought, leaving more of their working memory available to critically think and problem solve.

A few more points about briefings. In the cockpit of an airliner, briefings also occur at several points within the flight, not just in the beginning shortly after the crew comes together. They are woven into the cockpit checklist and are part of normal operating procedures. Additional briefings typically occur just prior to takeoff, prior to the start of an approach to landing, and prior to any emergency or abnormal landing (time permitting). The point to make here is that these briefings tend to be more focused on a particular phase or task of the operation and build off the initial more comprehensive crew briefing that sets the overall tone. For example, just prior to takeoff, with all checklists complete, operating procedures call for the pilot flying to conduct a short briefing of intended actions; this tends to be very succinct in most cases. It generally covers the initial heading or direction the aircraft will fly, the initial altitude the aircraft will climb to, and the runway that will be used if an emergency return is necessary. It may sound something like this:

> *"OK, we will fly heading 220 and climb to 5000. If we have an emergency, we will plan on runway one-seven left. Any questions?"*

This same idea of inserting succinct, task-focused briefings at key points throughout the shift is a good one. For example, an RN may brief another RN just prior to entering a patient's room to perform a complicated dressing change:

"OK, we'll use sterile technique for Mr. Smith's dressing change. After the old dressing is removed, I'll don sterile gloves. I'll definitely need you to open dressing supplies and place them on our sterile field. We'll need pads for the irrigation. He's been medicated for pain, but let's be gentle when we reposition him. This is very unpleasant for him, so let's move rapidly while maintaining good technique. Do you have questions? Have I missed anything?"

When conducting a briefing, it is important to use language that is team oriented. Words like "we," "us," and "let's" should be emphasized wherever possible and are always preferable to words that separate, such as "you" or "I." Notice the language in the briefing above: *let's, we, we'll, our.* This is inclusive language and works to say subconsciously, "Hey, we're in this together." It is also absolutely imperative that team leaders don't assume ownership of team members through their language. When I was a pilot, I would occasionally hear some captains telling stories in the crew lounge about a particular flight. When doing so they would say "My F/O [first officer] did this"; or "I told my F/O to do that." "My?" This drove me crazy. This language does not facilitate team-work; it implies intense authority and subservience. I NEVER used this language as a captain. Unfortunately, I frequently hear this on nursing units and throughout healthcare. Physicians will say "my nurse." Nurses will say "my aide," and so on. Words have meanings, both implied and explicit, and words that imply ownership of people have no place in the team glossary.

To wrap things up, here is an example of an RN briefing a nursing assistant at the start of a day. The RN has received handoff report and now wants to set the proper tone for teamwork and effective communication during the shift. The briefing will cover only one patient for the purposes of demonstration. See if you think it has the attributes of a good briefing and creates a shared mental model:

Hi, Mary, how are you doing this morning? It's good to be working with you again.

Before we go through the briefing checklist for each patient, I want to cover a few items, OK? First, let's be sure that whatever we do today, we follow hospital policies and procedures. It's very important that we don't take shortcuts. If we feel pressure to do that because of time constraints, we should stop and ask for help. It's imperative that we keep our patients safe first and foremost.

Also, while we work together today, if you see anything that concerns you or doesn't make sense, please speak up. I'm not perfect and I may miss things, so please let me know if you find something in your assessment that we both need to be aware of; it doesn't matter how small or unimportant it may seem. In fact, I expect you to speak up and tell me what your concerns are—always. OK?

Now let's go through the briefing checklist for each patient. With Mrs. Jones, since she had surgery yesterday, our focus will be on postoperative care. Our main goal is to control her pain early on and keep her comfortable. Also, let's make sure that we get her out of bed ambulating around the unit at least twice during our shift and that she is coughing and deep breathing. If we can do that, I think we will have accomplished something with her today, and this will help us move her one step closer to discharge. I will do my complete assessment when I round and begin passing meds. After you get vital signs and assist her a.m. care, let me know if you need my assistance getting her up.

Do you have any questions, Mary?

OK, thanks; let's have a good shift today."

Inviting Participation

As a first officer at the airlines, one of the things I remember was the consistent use of the briefing by the captain. More importantly, part of that briefing was the distinct invitation by the captain for me to participate in the process. Some did this better than others, of course, but the theme was consistent. My participation was not only requested—it was expected. For example, many captains would say something like this:

*"I'm not perfect, and from time to time I'll miss something or make a mistake.
If you see anything at all that concerns you, something doesn't seem right, or you see
me doing something that doesn't make sense, please speak up. As a matter of fact, I
expect you to speak up. OK?"*

Recall that this strategy was used in our previous med–surg briefing example. It seems
rather simple. It seems obvious that if something is wrong, someone will speak up and bring
it to the attention of the team or the team leader. But history suggests otherwise. Aviation
archives are replete with airline disasters in which someone on the flight deck knew something bad could or was about to happen, yet they did not bring that information forward,
either at all, or forcefully enough (think about UAL Flight 173 in Chapter 1). Requesting
participation and making it an expectation is a team-building strategy. **It must be openly
stated again and again**. Team leaders can never assume that team members get it when it
comes to speaking up. This expectation and behavior needs constant reinforcement.

Healthcare team leaders, whether a surgeon in the OR, a charge nurse on a nursing unit,
or an RN briefing a nursing assistant, must set a tone that fosters open communication.
A simple but effective way to do this is to openly invite people to speak up when they see
something that concerns them, no matter what, or as in the briefing example, no matter how
small or unimportant it may seem. It should be stated every time the team is together, and it
must be made clear that rank, title, or status in the organization should not prohibit questioning the actions of an individual or the team as a whole.

As an airline captain, I continued using basically the same script described previously, but
I added verbiage that communicated the point that the most important thing was feedback.
I didn't care whether crew members were mistaken in their concerns, and I didn't care
whether their feedback turned out to be incorrect. The important point was that they were
bringing their assessments and concerns forward. Of course, the expectation is that a team
member is critically thinking, but I never wanted anyone not to speak up for fear of being
wrong. A good line for a team leader to use here is: "I'd much rather you speak up about

something that turns out to be nothing than say nothing about a concern that turns out to be something." ◆

As nurse team leaders, we must remember to walk the walk and not just make empty promises because it sounds good superficially. Asking for feedback is half of the equation; the other half is receiving it well and really demonstrating that you are pleased when a team member raises a question or concern in the interest of safety, even if it turns out to be nothing.

Evaluate the following true case:

A nurse entered a patient's room during start-of-shift rounds. The patient was in pain and wanted IV push Dilaudid. The nurse checked the medication adminis-tration record and determined that the patient was due for the medication. She administered the drug and shortly after the patient's blood pressure (BP) bottomed out. Confusion ensued. A code was called and the patient responded well, although he was transferred to a step-down unit for observation. The RN later looked at the vital signs that were taken by the nursing assistant (NA) just prior to rounds. The BP was recorded as 88/50, which was a change from previous readings for this patient. The RN asked the NA about this. She stated that while she noticed the BP was low, she thought that the nurse would see it, so she didn't say anything.

Might the outcome have been different had the RN briefed the NA at the start of the shift, and that briefing included an explicit invitation to speak up with any concerns, no matter how small?

Questions

When you pull the gas-powered lawnmower out of the shed for the first cut of the year, do you immediately start pulling on the cord hoping the engine will start? No. You must first press the little plunger that primes the system with gas. The same is true with teams. As a nurse leader on the unit, you have to prime the patient care team for communication.

Gaffney et al. describe "asking questions" as a simple but effective strategy to initiate the flow of information.[24] This means that after you greet members of your team at the start of a shift, and you prepare for the work ahead, casually ask a few open-ended questions. When the person responds, you listen. Then you will respond and they will listen. It is a great strategy to prime or reinforce the process of talking to each other and exchanging information. Although it is good if questions are related to operational matters, the subject is much less important than the question itself. It is also not a bad idea to have preplanned or stock questions that you can draw from.

What do you think?

You are an RN in charge of the care for a group of seven patients. One patient has a BP that is uncharacteristically low when compared to his overall trend. You recheck the pressure and there is no change; the patient is otherwise fine and presents no unusual findings. You decide to hold the patient's BP medications and consult with the physician when he arrives on the unit for rounds about an hour later. You are completely comfortable with this plan, but when you inform the LPN you are working with today about your decision, you punctuate it with the question, "What do you think about that?" You want the people on your team to get into the habit of communicating their observations and concerns to you. A great way to facilitate that process is simply to ask them what they think when the opportunity presents itself. Doing this produces several positive outcomes. In this case, the LPN will feel valued as part of the team because you demonstrated an interest in his or her opinion. It also reinforces expectations to participate in the decision-making process.

Soaring to Success

You may be thinking, "What if the LPN disagrees with my decision when I ask for input?" That's fine. Remember, as the leader, you make the final call, but as we have discussed, decisions are best when you have the team participating. Listen to the rationale for disagreement. If it does not change the decision, thank them for their input and move forward. If information is offered that you did not consider or were not aware of, you can reevaluate your plan, which ultimately strengthens the decision. It is also important to remember that while this is an effective tactic to establish team communication, it should be used strategically and only when time permits.

Setting the Acknowledgment Expectation

Finally, another important team-building behavior is making it clear that all members of the team will receive acknowledgment when they offer feedback or have a question. That acknowledgment can be verbal or nonverbal, but it must occur in some form. Let's go back to the cockpit. Leaders in the cockpit will set the behavioral expectation that when someone speaks, either by making a statement of fact or asking a direct question, the crew member on the receiving end will acknowledge. This behavior is modeled by the leader so that in time, team members feel like something is wrong if communications are not actively acknowledged. Captains often say something such as:

"If you say something to me and I don't respond, say it again until I do."

Remember that communication is a loop, and this loop must be closed.[24] This behavioral expectation is essential for several reasons, the first being that it takes the guesswork out of communication. It is not a pleasant feeling to impart what you consider to be important information only to wonder whether the receiver heard what you said. Think about how you feel when your spouse does this to you. It is often the cause of many marital disputes. It is important to emphasize that an acknowledgement response should convey genuine receipt of the information imparted. Sometimes communication can be acknowledged verbally, but receivers' body language and the nature of their response indicates that information may not have been heard or understood. If acknowledgements are partial or ambiguous, the sender must clarify to close the communication loop.

Setting the acknowledgment expectation makes it acceptable to repeat things or ask, "Did you hear what I just said?" It's not rudeness; It's just a technique to ensure effective communication in the operational environment. Nurses frequently share information with physicians as they quickly round on the unit, but often acknowledgments are absent or incomplete. The same is true when patients and families offer observations or questions to nurses and other clinicians; acknowledgments may not occur or be less than optimal. Nurses and physicians would do well to set the acknowledgment expectation at the outset and live by it, just as pilots do.

Readback

One very simple tool to use is the readback. The readback is often used by nurses to close the communication loop after receiving telephone orders or critical lab values. But why stop there? It is a good idea to use the readback for a multitude of situations on the unit. Here is a simple example. You have a patient who needs a chest tube drainage set changed, and then the tube needs to be switched from continuous suction to water seal. You are busy with another patient, so another nurse offers to do it for you. As the nurse starts walking away to complete the task, you say, "Can you give me a readback?" The nurse reads it back, confirming the correct patient and the instructions. If you set that expectation as the leader by asking for a readback, people come to expect it. Soon, you will find that the receiver of information will say, "Let me give you a readback" if you forget to ask for one. Now that is a unit culture that closes the loop on communication.

Another very important reason that acknowledgments are critical to safety is they can identify when someone is incapacitated, fatigued, or not engaged. There are times that pilots and nurses can lose focus, or become ill or fatigued. Usually in these situations the first sign is to stop communicating. No acknowledgments may mean that someone is in trouble and needs to be rescued. When someone on the healthcare team does not acknowledge communication, it must be investigated further, and the culture must support this behavior.

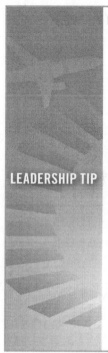

LEADERSHIP TIP

Let's review team building and leadership strategies covered in Chapters 4 and 5:

- Use interpersonal skills

- Greet team members; engage them in conversation

- Actively listen via eye contact, body language, and verbal affirmation

- Set the tone (polite, professional, and by the book)

- Use the leadership grid to balance focus on people vs. task for clinical situations

- Brief your team early on

- Establish a mental model; share it in the briefing

- Invite participation; make it an expectation

- Involve team members by asking them, "What do you think?"

- Acknowledge all communication; make it an expectation

References

1. Kern, A.T., *Controlling Pilot Error: Culture, Environment, & CRM. 2001,* New York: McGraw Hill. p. 75–77.

2. World Health Organization. *WHO Surgical Safety Checklist.* 2009 [cited 6/14/2010]; Available from: *http://whqlibdoc.who.int/publications/2009/9789241598590_eng_Checklist.pdf.*

3. Haynes, A.B., T.G. Weiser, W.R. Berry, et al. A surgical safety checklist to reduce morbidity and mortality in a global population. *New England Journal of Medicine, 2009. 360*: p. 491–499.

4. Winters, D.D., A.P. Gurses, H. Lehmann, and et al. Clinical review: Checklists—translating evidence into practice. *Critical Care, 2009. 13*(6).

5. Sutcliffe, K.M., E. Lewton, and M.M. Rosenthal, Communication failures: an insidious contributor to medical mishaps. *Academic Medicine, 2004. 79*: p. 186–194.

6. Lingard, L., S. Espin, S. Whyte, et al., Communication failures in the operating room: An observational classification of recurrent types and effects. *Quality and Safety in Health Care, 2004. 13*: p. 330–334.

7. Decker, S., *The Field Guide to Human Error Investigations.* 2002, Burlington, VT: Ashgate.

8. Musson, D.M., and R.L. Helmreich. Team training and resource management in health care: Current issues and future directions. *Harvard Health Policy Review, 2004. 5*(1): p. 25–35.

9. Medicine, I.O. *To Err is Human: Building a Safer Health Care System,* L.T. Kohn, J. Corrigan, and M.S. Donaldson, Editors. 2000, Washington, DC: National Academic Press.

10. Gawande, A. *The Checklist Manifesto.* 2009, New York: Metropolitan. p. 156.

11. Pratt, S.D., S. Mann, M. Salisbury, et al. Impact of CRM-based team training on obstetric outcomes and clinicians' safety attitudes. *Joint Commission Journal of Quality and Patient Safety 2007. 33*: p. 720–725.

12. Helmreich, R.L., J.A. Wilhelm, S.E. Gregorich, T.R. Chidester. Preliminary results from the evaluation of cockpit resource management training: performance rating of flight crews. *Aviation, Space, and Environmental Medicine, 1990. 61*: p. 576–9.

13. Endsley, M.R. Theoretical Underpinnings of Situational Awareness: A Critical Review in *Situational Awareness Analysis and Measurement,* M.R. Endsley and D.J. Garland, Editors. 2000, Mahwah, NJ: Lawrence Erlbaum and Associates.

14. Pope, J. Checklists: Guideposts often ignored. *Accident Prevention, 1991. 48*(5).

15. Flight Safety Foundation. Approach and Landing Accident Reduction in *Flight Safety Digest.* 2000, August–November.

16. Reason, J., *Managing the Risks of Organizational Accidents.* 1998, Aldershot, United Kingdom: Ashgate.

17. Klein, G., *Sources of Power: How People Make Decisions.* 1999, Cambridge, MA: MIT Press.

18. Fiore, S., M. Rosen, E. Salas, S. Burke, and F. Jentsch. Processes in Complex Team Problem-solving: Parsing and Defining the Theoretical Problem Space in *Marcrocognition in Teams,* M. Letsky, et al., Editors. 2008, Burlington, VT: Ashgate.

19. McComb, S., Shared Mental Models and their Convergence, in *Macrorecognition in Teams*, M. Letsky, et al., Editors. 2008, Burlington, VT: Ashgate.

20. Cannon-Bowers, J., E. Salas, and S. Converse. Shared Mental Models in Expert Team Decision Making, in *Individual and Group Decision Making: Current Issues*, N.J. Castellan, Editor. 1993, Hillsdale, NJ: Lawrence Erlbaum. p. 221–246.

21. Bordetsky, A. and S. Hutchins, Plug-and-Play Testbed for Collaboration in the Global Information Grid in *Macrorecognition in Teams*, M. Letsky, et al., Editors. 2008, Burlington, VT: Ashgate.

22. Lagadec, P., *Preventing Chaos in a Crisis: Strategies for prevention, control, and damage limitation.* 1993, New York: McGraw Hill.

23. Sun-tzu, *The Art of War,* ed. R.D. Sawyer. 1994, New York: Barnes and Noble.

24. Gaffney, F.A., S.W. Harden, and R. Seddon, *Crew Resource Management: The Flight Plan for Lasting Change in Patient Safety.* 2005, Marblehead, MA: HcPro.

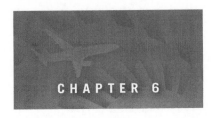

CHAPTER 6

Followership: Putting an End to "Hint-and-Hope" Communication

In Chapters 4 and 5, we discussed how crew resource management (CRM) promotes leadership styles that are participatory in nature and that an effective leader sets a tone where all members of the team feel free to express concerns regarding what the team is about to do. Participatory leaders empower team members in such a way that they feel compelled to speak up when they have concerns about operational safety and use specific strategies and tools to facilitate this type of atmosphere. It is clear that in the cockpit a captain can make better decisions when the flight crew is engaged and providing feedback. The same is true in healthcare.

Team leaders, whether physicians or nurses, will make better decisions about patient care when authority gradients, hierarchy, and fear are removed from the equation, and all members of the team are engaged in the process. This chapter examines the engagement of team members in decision making, another key component in effective team communication.

Followership

Picture yourself at a conference sitting in an audience of fellow nurses and the speaker proclaims that "nurses must learn to become better followers." How would you respond? You would not be alone if you found this statement repugnant. When I engage in discussion with groups of frontline nurses on the concept of followership, an expression of distaste initially appears on many faces in the crowd. Fair enough. Ultimately, we want nurses who are leaders, not followers. To many, the word "follower" implies that someone blithely stands by waiting to be told what to do, ready to carry out orders handed down from above. However, as we explore the concept further within the context of CRM, it is clear that this description of a follower is not even remotely accurate.

Followership is an active process and does not imply passivity. Tony Kern, author of *Controlling Pilot Error* (2002), says that assertiveness is a mandatory prerequisite to effective followership. Not everyone can be in charge. When team members begin to jockey for position and power, performance suffers. National Aeronautics and Space Administration (NASA) research confirms this point. When considering personality profile assessments for astronaut candidate selection, an overly competitive interpersonal orientation can be linked to poor team performance.[1]

However, because one person is ultimately the decision maker does not imply that followers take a hands-off approach. On the contrary, effective followers feel a sense of responsibility and pride in team performance and see themselves as an integral part of the decision-making process. They assume ownership for the quality and safety of team decisions and never sit idly by while their team proceeds with a course of action that poses unacceptable risks. Stated simply, if you are on a team, you must provide the team leader with precise, specific, and timely feedback that is both accurate and honest.

Being a follower requires that you use your brain, that you critically think through situations, and that you are prepared to communicate that information regardless of someone's rank or title in the organization.

This is the essence of inquiry and advocacy: assertive behaviors essential to followership. Inquiry means that you question everything and do not accept things at face value. You are skeptical and seek to confirm any operating premise held by the team. Advocacy means that you are prepared to bring forward an alternative course of action, even if it is contrary to what is accepted. The following are examples of inquiry:

- A nurse caring for a septic patient in an intensive care unit (ICU) queries a physician as to why a particular antibiotic was discontinued.

- When discussing a frail, elderly patient during handoff report, a nurse asks the charge nurse why the patient has not been placed on high-risk fall precautions.

The following is an example of advocacy:

Two residents and a registered nurse are gathered at a patient's bedside on a medical–surgical unit preparing to do an incision and drainage of a large foot wound. The patient is draped and everyone is ready to proceed. The residents ask the nurse to inject 50 mg Demerol and 25 Versed IV push. The nurse knows this is considered "moderate sedation" according to policy and requires specifically trained personnel and cardiac monitoring. One of the residents tells the nurse to get a heart monitor from the crash cart and just give the medication; the other nods in agreement. The nurse tells them both that this is not protocol and she cannot proceed. The nurse then calls the appropriate personnel to the floor to administer the drug and monitor the patient per hospital policy.

Kelly's Model

Figure 6.1 references an adaptation of Kelly's Model of Followership.[2, 3] In this model, there are four quadrants created by the intersection of two lines, one horizontal line that represents degrees of activity or engagement, and a vertical line that shows the degree of critical thinking that occurs. The model places followers on a quadrant based on the degree to which they possess these attributes, indicating effective or ineffective followership.

Soaring to Success

FIGURE
6.1

Followership Model

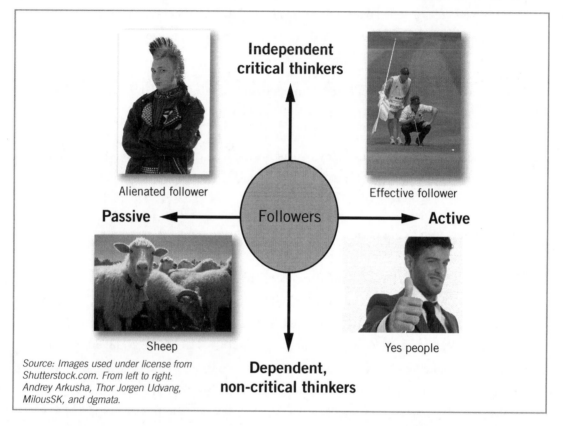

Source: Images used under license from Shutterstock.com. From left to right: Andrey Arkusha, Thor Jorgen Udvang, MilousSK, and dgmata.

In the bottom quadrant you see sheep. Sheep are not inherently dangerous as followers, but they offer nothing to the team. They think of no new ideas, and they are not actively involved in the process of decision making. Basically, sheep take up space. Perhaps you can think of characters and faces that fit this description.

The bottom right quadrant offers us the "yes" person. "Yes" people do not represent the kind of follower we want in the cockpit or on the healthcare team. They are not critical thinkers, yet they are active in the decision-making process. They support whatever the leader decides to do, perpetually bobbing their heads up and down in agreement. This makes them dangerous, for if the team leader or the team as a whole is about to do something unsafe, you can bet the "yes" person will be onboard. "Yes" people are great for the team leader's ego, but bad for operational safety. Consider the following case:

> *A nurse on a medical–surgical unit is caring for a patient following abdominal surgery. The patient is receiving a standard Dilaudid patient-controlled anesthesia (PCA) protocol that includes a continuous background infusion of 1 mg per hour in addition to the PCA dosing that the patient controls every 15 minutes. Information given in handoff report indicates that the patient has been somnolent, falling asleep throughout the day, and has been sluggish when ambulating.*
>
> *Through assessment, the nurse notes that while bowel sounds are present, gastrointestinal function has been slow to return. The patient has mild respiratory congestion that clears with coughing, but is not progressing well with postoperative inspiratory exercises. The patient does not appear to be in distress but frequently pushes the PCA pump button. While standing at the front desk writing an order sheet, the surgical resident tells the nurse that he is extending the continuous infusion for an additional 24 hours because the patient stated that she has been in "a lot of pain." Eager to please the resident, the nurse nods in agreement and says "OK, great."*
>
> *Is there basic critical thinking going on here on the part of this nurse? If there is, how could she stand silent and not offer feedback to the physician about the decision to continue IV pain medication for a patient who is oversedated and not reaching expected postoperative milestones? You can see that the "yes" person is not an effective follower and places the patient at risk. They should be retrained or removed from the team.*

In the upper left quadrant we have the recalcitrant alienated follower. This person is a great critical thinker. They are smart and many times have the answers the team is looking for. The problem here is that the alienated follower will not participate in the decision-making process because he or she has issues with the team, with the leader of the team, or the organization as a whole. The alienated follower can become so disenfranchised that he or she may knowingly, through their inaction, help the team fail. This can also be a dangerous situation.

Let me illustrate. I was once flying with a captain who was perhaps one of the most obnoxious individuals I have ever met. I couldn't stand him. He was rude, a know-it-all, and treated all of his first officers with little respect. On this night he was flying the aircraft executing an instrument approach procedure (referencing flight instruments only, not the ground) in steady rain. I noticed that he failed to press what is called an autopilot mode button. Pressing this button allows the autopilot to capture something called the glide path, which starts the aircraft smoothly descending toward the runway. I saw him forget to press the button. I thought to myself, "All right, you blowhard, I'm gonna sit back and watch you make this mistake. Maybe you'll be humbled." So, I just watched and said nothing. As the aircraft failed to descend, the captain became completely confused. He hesitated and then disengaged the autopilot and began flying the aircraft by hand, but as he did, our approach became very unstable. Our smooth descent became a series of small dives and level-offs with unpleasant fluctuations in speed. He eventually got it under control. After we landed, he continued to mumble to himself and make excuses about what happened; he wasn't acting so cocky anymore. Of course, what I did, or failed to do, was the real problem. I was a conscientious pilot and always supported the captain of the ship while speaking up when I needed to. Yet on this night, I allowed myself to become an alienated follower. I sat there and relegated operational safety to delighting in this captain's failure, which unfortunately was the team's failure, and it was my failure. There is no doubt that the passengers felt the aircraft lurch and descend; it clearly was not pleasant for them.

I vowed I would never allow that situation occur again, and I didn't. The same is true in nursing. Let's suppose those passengers were patients, and I was an ICU nurse instead of a first officer in an airplane. What if I sat by and allowed a physician to order the wrong drug on a patient, not pointing out the mistake because I had an axe to grind with him. That would be unconscionable. This is an extreme example, but alienated followers do exist, and their intelligence, coupled with lack of participation, can be subtle and dangerous.

One more point about the alienated follower. While conducting a CRM session for nurses I asked the following question, "What would you do if you saw a physician about to do something that was going to cause harm to a patient?" A nurse confidently said, "I would tell him to stop." I then said, "What if he or she ignored you and continued?" What the nurse said next astounded me. "Hey, I told him. It's on them at that point, but I would document what occurred." This is an alienated follower. Needless to say, from the patient's point of view this approach is patently unacceptable.

Effective followers follow a simple rule: If you see it, you own it. You cannot disengage and allow someone on the team to press forward with actions that you believe to be unsafe because he or she is rude or will not listen. ◆

Finally, we come to the effective follower. This is what CRM espouses. In the upper right quadrant of Kelly's model, you will see a picture of a professional golfer and caddy. Caddies represent effective followers. Caddies carry the clubs, hold the flags, clean the balls, walk the course, and pull out the clubs from the bag. In addition, caddies calculate yardage, offer advice on what club to use, offer suggestions on how the ball will break when putting, and assist with overall strategy on the golf course. They are critically thinking and active. These are the professionals we

---

◆ Sidebar 6.1

Followership and trust relationships

The level of followers' trust in a leader influences the choice to follow a leader and practice good followership. Trust between followers and team leaders builds on norms of reciprocity and civic engagement.[4]

In general, people trust others either because these others have acted in favorable ways in the past or they can be expected to act favorably in the future.[5] Organizational theorists recognize that treatment with respect and dignity is the most important predictor of trustworthiness. In other words, people find authorities to be trustworthy because those authorities treat them politely. A leader being respectful is a better predictor of trust by followers than agreement with the leader's decisions or even sharing power with the leader in decision making.[6]

want on our healthcare teams, whether those teams consist of five people in an operating room or two nurses working together on a medical–surgical unit.

So far, we have discussed followership with regard to feedback and explained that it should be specific, timely, accurate, and honest. There are some questions to consider now: First, how do we provide such feedback, and what is the best technique or tool for doing so? Second, what do we do if we provide specific, honest, accurate, and timely feedback, but we are not heard? In the next section, we will explore these questions.

Hint and Hope: What NOT to Do

Followership requires directness. There can be no beating around the bush, especially in high-risk, complex settings such as airplanes and acute care hospitals. There is a term that I was first exposed to as a pilot sitting in a CRM class called "hint and hope." Hinting and hoping occurs when someone speaks cryptically about a concern, then waits for the receiver to decipher the code and act on that concern. Unfortunately, hinting and hoping is a suboptimal form of communication that almost always fails. To illustrate, let's look at an airline scenario.

On August 2, 1985, Delta Air Lines Flight 191 was on final approach to Dallas/Fort Worth International Airport. As the jet continued its descent to the runway, the copilot became concerned about an ominous looking thunderstorm directly ahead. He did not want to fly through it and was clearly not comfortable with what they were about to do. The copilot attempted to communicate his concerns to the captain, and did so by simply pointing out the fact that lightning was shooting out from the bottom of the cloud formation. He did this twice, but the captain's response was delayed and dismissive. The copilot was hinting at his serious reservations about the safety of the flight by pointing out the presence of lightning. He then hoped the captain would catch on, become engaged, and steer the aircraft away from danger. It didn't work. Delta 191 encountered severe wind shear at low altitude and crashed short of the runway. One hundred thirty-five people were killed, including one person on the ground. The pilots did not survive.

In a better scenario, hint-and-hope communication could be replaced by direct, specific statements about the danger and its potential effect on a safe outcome. There is no specific formula here; all that is required is to just say it out loud—be direct and to the point. Consider the following statement for this scenario: "That looks unsafe ahead. I'm concerned about low level wind shear. Let's consider aborting this approach." With this communication there is no doubt about the concern and what is on the mind of the copilot. At the very least, this statement should engage the captain so that further discussion could take place. Now let's move to nursing and expand on this discussion. ◆

> ◆ Sidebar 6.2
> ## Social hierarchy, control, and CRM adoption
>
> Effective CRM requires a rethinking of the utility of social hierarchies traditionally found in medicine. One study found that only 55% of surgeons rejected steep hierarchies (determined by whether they thought junior team members should question the decisions of senior team members). In contrast, 94% of airline crew members preferred the flat hierarchies that encourage communication and better followership.[7] It may be that one of the larger obstacles to overcome in the adoption of CRM concepts is the resistance by medical team physician leaders, who are concerned about losing autonomy and authority.[8] Conversely, nurses are typically quick to embrace human factors concepts, including organizational structures that facilitate communication.[9]

Hint and Hope: The Way Nurses Communicate?

I was encouraged when I discovered the work of Leonard, Graham, and Bonacum, which discusses the "hint-and-hope" phenomenon as it applies to clinicians.[10] They suggest that this style of communication has long been the norm in healthcare and is "fraught with risk." Nurses traditionally have received little or no training in how to communicate patient information to physicians effectively, especially when the clinical picture is inconclusive and there are not indisputable signs of patient deterioration. It is simple to relay the fact that a patient has crushing chest pain, but quite another to cogently piece together subtle changes and vague complaints in a convincing fashion.

Also complicating the matter is the fact that nurses may view approaching or calling a physician with trepidation and hesitancy. The paradigm has traditionally been one that elevates the status of physicians and places greater value on their time. It is not uncommon to hear a nurse use the phrase, "I'm sorry to bother you," as a preface to conveying patient information. Nurses may then feel rushed and pressured in their communication, perceiving that they have only a small window of opportunity to state their case. Consider too that nurses have been told repeatedly by all levels of hospital administration that physicians are their customers, implying that the overriding objective is to satisfy physicians. This undermines collegiality and hinders open communication when the situation calls for advocating a course of action in direct opposition to what a physician intends. Imagine this situation being replicated on an airplane: The copilots are employed by the airline but the captains are not, viewed only as visitors by the organization? What would be the net effect on team communication if the copilots were told that the captain's satisfaction was their responsibility? I would not fly that airline.

Fear and intimidation also challenge effective followership. Often nurses will fail to fully convey serious concerns or information regarding the status of their patients in the face of intimidating or dismissive communication styles on the part of physicians (medical team leaders). In fact, nurses may assume the hint-and-hope mode at even the anticipation of a difficult encounter with a physician. More than 2,000 nurses and pharmacists were survey by the Institute for Safe Medication Practices in 2003, and 49% of those surveyed indicated that past intimidation altered their handling of order clarifications or questions. In other words, if a nurse expects that he or she will experience a negative encounter (raised voice intonations, yelling, abrupt rebukes, profanity, and sarcastic responses), there is an increased likelihood the nurse will hint and hope when initiating the communication. Worse yet, the encounter may be avoided altogether.

I have often felt that the famed and ubiquitous sticky note left on the chart by nurses for physicians to find and hopefully read is nothing more than a form of hint-and-hope communication: It is rarely effective and often not considered. ◆

Let's now look at some tools to assist nurses in practicing effective followership.

◆ Sidebar 6.3

Communication and error

Inadequate communication is one of the most researched causes of preventable medical errors.[11] Because each caregiver has a unique perspective and professional culture—and clinical disciplines train separately—it is understandable why miscommunication is a common and major contributor to medical errors.[12–14] However, CRM does not mean that one suspends all cultural rules for communication. There is ample evidence that an unbounded openness in communication can create problems across necessary role boundaries and in intercultural settings.[15] One of the important actions taken by the team leader to encourage followership will be to specify what the expectation is for communication for effective problem solving and patient safety.

Carol has been a nurse for 10 months and is caring for a postsurgical patient, Miss Gibson, who is experiencing increased pain at the surgical site and a consistent low-grade fever. In addition to these findings, Carol thinks the patient is less energetic than the previous two days. Laboratory findings show a slight increase in the white blood cell count, though still within the high normal range. Dr. Smith, Miss Gibson's surgeon, is rounding through the unit at a steady pace. He appears focused on seeing his patients and returning to the OR. Dr. Smith is usually all business and is known for his direct responses.

Carol is concerned about her patient. She isn't sure whether her assessment is significant but has been caring for Miss Gibson all week and is not entirely comfortable with the clinical picture. She understands that her findings may be within the realm of a normal recovery. She also understands that her findings could be early signs of a postoperative infection. In this case early intervention and therapy is critical to a favorable outcome for the patient. She wants to inform Dr. Smith, but knows that he doesn't like to be bothered for trivial matters. Carol is a good nurse and has been steadily developing confidence, but she possesses the normal doubts that accompany any fledgling clinician. What should she say to Dr. Smith?

This is a classic example of what nurses experience frequently at the point of care. For some, being assertive and providing specific feedback, even in the face of a nonreceptive team leader like Dr. Smith, is not difficult. For others it is a tall order. Perhaps Carol will "hint" and say, "Dr. Smith, did you notice anything different about Miss Gibson today?" then stand there "hoping" that Dr. Smith will engage and ask for more information. This is unlikely given the fact that this physician is not known for extended conversation and interpersonal warmth. Indeed, if Dr. Smith responds by saying "No, I didn't when I was there earlier this morning," and then walks off, the conversation could end at that point and the chance for real information exchange is lost. If Carol's findings are representative of an early postoperative infection, most likely precious time will be lost until the signs and symptoms are much more pronounced.

Carol can serve herself and the patient much better by remembering to be specific about what she **sees**, what her concerns are, and what she wants. "Dr. Smith, Miss Gibson has maintained a temp of 99.8, she has a slight elevation in her WBCs, she's having pain at the incision and seems lethargic as compared to yesterday. I'm **concerned** that she may be developing a postoperative infection. I **want** you to reevaluate her before you leave the unit." This is specific, direct, and concise and has within it a requested course of action. There is no doubt what Carol's assessment is and what she wants—there is no "hinting and hoping."

LEADERSHIP TIP

The 3Ws are an excellent tool for use in dynamic, real-time situations in which feedback must be formulated and delivered promptly to achieve a safe outcome. In the preceding example, Carol used the 3Ws.

- What I see

- What I am concerned about

- What I want

Effective followership means that there is an inherent responsibility to speak up and bring perceived problems that affect safety to the table so discrepancies can be resolved. Leonard et al. discuss the use of standardized communication tools to ensure effective communication and feedback and advocate the use of SBAR as a way to accomplish this:[10]

- **S**ituation

- **B**ackground

- **A**ssessment

- **R**ecommendation

This is an excellent CRM-based tool that has its roots in the military. The use of SBAR in healthcare has been encouraging with positive outcomes for both patients and staff in several high-risk areas such as the operating room, emergency room, and intensive care.[10, 16, 17] Without entering into a comprehensive discussion about SBAR (you can find many sources for more information on this topic), the overarching point is that a planned and/or standardized communication method provides specific feedback in a succinct and timely manner, offering a suggested course of action.

I advocate the 3Ws because of its simplicity. Simply answer the questions and you can easily put your thoughts together in a statement that is specific, direct, and concise. Whether a nurse chooses to use the 3Ws or SBAR, planning and standardizing critical communication will serve to avoid the classic hint-and-hope trap.

What If I'm Still Not Heard? Assertive Communication Tools

Several years ago, I was flying as a young first officer for a regional airline. It was barely light on a brisk December morning as the Saab 340 Airliner sat parked on the tarmac. The captain, whom I'll call Tom, sat in the left seat of the aircraft completing his preflight inspection of the flight deck. I sat in the right seat and began to inspect and set up my side of the cockpit. Just moments before, I had completed my external walk-around inspection (also called the preflight) of the aircraft. During my inspection, I used a flashlight to inspect the undercarriage of the plane because there was not yet enough daylight to provide adequate illumination for inspection. As I walked around the aircraft in the cold morning air, I noticed that a wintery mix began to fall lightly from the sky. There was some snow mixed with sleet. After all of our cockpit checks were complete, I took note of the fact that the wintery mix was still lightly falling. I tuned in the airport automated weather, which was now reporting snow and ice pellets. At this point I heard the ground crew query the captain via radio regarding our intentions for de-icing. When asked whether we wanted to be deiced, Tom replied, "Negative." It was possible to see a limited portion of the right wing from the cockpit, but it was still too dark to get a clear picture of whether the wing was becoming contaminated with snow and ice, an absolute danger that can spell disaster for an aircraft when attempting to gain the required lift to takeoff. The captain's decision was cause for some concern, but I rationalized that deicing would not be required as the precipitation was falling at a slow enough rate that there was unlikely to be any build up before we took off. Tom was an older fellow and was unpredictable in his moods. He did things his way and let you know it if he thought you were asking too many questions. Many times during the month (airlines sometimes pair pilots together for a month at a time), I had brought things to Tom's attention regarding procedural steps that were missed. He corrected the issues but became very agitated. I chose at this point to say nothing to Tom about the deicing situation.

We now had all passengers on board, both engines running, and we were ready to begin our taxi to the runway. Outside the cockpit I could see that the rate of precipitation was getting heavier. This was starting to concern me; you could hear the faint snap of ice pellets hitting the skin and windshield of the airplane over the engine noise and I began to picture the thin layer of snow and ice building up on the wing and tail surfaces. I did not like this at all. My heart started pounding as I reviewed in my mind the string of airline accidents caused by ice buildup on takeoff. As the aircraft began to taxi, I said to the captain, "Man, it's really coming down out there" (hint and hope). Tom said nothing. At that moment we taxied close to a splash of light from the large spotlights that illuminated the tarmac at night. I looked out of the window and backward and got a good look at a small section of the wing. There was snow and ice clearly building up on the wing surface. Tom just kept on taxiing the aircraft and began calling for the taxi checklist. It was a horrible predicament. It felt completely wrong and extremely uncomfortable to continue, but I knew Tom would blow his stack if I began to push the issue. This was a defining moment. I recognized a trigger, a red flag. That feeling of extreme discomfort with what we were about to do, coupled with an acute awareness of the fact that it defied all policy and sound judgment, pushed me over the edge. I immediately and with conviction employed the four-step assertive communication tool that I learned in CRM training. It went like this:

1. **Get attention:** "Tom [with emphasis]."

2. **State the problem:** "I'm really not comfortable with this. Its coming down pretty hard out there and I can see that there is significant contamination on the wing."

3. **Offer a plan:** "I suggest we go back to the gate and get deiced."

4. **Pose a question, get resolution:** "Do you agree with me?"

To say that Tom was not happy was a colossal understatement. He yelled an expletive and pushed hard on the brakes of the aircraft (too hard in my opinion). The aircraft lurched forward as we came to a stop. He looked at me and started muttering more profanity. But what he did next was key. He squeezed the transmit button and told the ground controller that we were returning to the gate to be deiced. At that moment, I didn't care what Tom said to me or how he treated me. I got what I wanted and operational safety was preserved. That feeling of acute discomfort coupled with tachycardia, dry mouth, and sweaty palms instantly subsided.

This is a true story with a good ending. Every pilot knows that taking off with ice and snow on the wings is unsafe and goes against all good decision making; no pilot would purposefully do so. Yet, here we were in a situation that unfolded in a way where we very easily could have done just that. From this experience it is easy to see that policies and regulations do not in and of themselves guarantee safe operations. On the contrary, it is the human response in the multitude of possible scenarios in everyday operations that makes or breaks operational safety.

Initially, I attempted the suboptimal hint-and-hope strategy. Making the comment, "Man, it's really coming down out there" accomplishes nothing and requires nothing from the captain. If Tom catches my hint and does what I want, then all is well. One could argue that it is effective to start with a hint and escalate from there as necessary. This strategy may be acceptable if:

1. You are aware that you are actually starting with a hint and fully prepared and ready to become more assertive if necessary

2. You are dealing with someone who has a participatory leadership style and is comfortable soliciting and receiving feedback

3. The situation is not time critical and there is sufficient time to move through the added steps, the back-and-forth communication

None of these things applied in this case. On the other hand, my comment about it "really coming down," though a hint, along with the obvious wintery mix falling at the airport should have been addressed by the captain, but it wasn't. He was not engaged, he didn't hear me, and he wasn't going to.

At its foundation, CRM programs teach the use of an **assertive communication tool to be used when it is absolutely necessary to achieve resolution among team members regarding safety.** The tool is simple and consists of the four steps outlined above. Let's apply the four-step assertive communication tool to the nursing domain.

Step 1

In Step 1, address individuals to get their attention. Start with their title (e.g., Dr. Jones). Sometimes, it may be necessary to strip away titles if you feel the situation is serious enough to warrant such a measure. If suddenly you call Dr. Jones by his first name, "Bill!" you will get his attention.

Step 2

In Step 2 the problem is stated. When doing so, it is good to preface your statement with the words, "I'm uncomfortable with ..." or "I'm concerned about ..." or some variation on that theme. This makes it clear that not only are you about to provide information, but also that you are deeply concerned about the situation or what the team is about to do.

After this preface, state the problem. It is very important to state the problem factually and concisely. It has been said that nurses communicate differently than physicians do. Nurses paint situations in great detail and may describe extraneous information not directly related to the main issue, sometimes referred to as the "building a watch instead of telling the time" phenomenon. It is generally thought that physicians as a group like the bottom line when communicating and get frustrated with too much detail. When looking at general tendencies among these professional groups, I would cautiously agree with that statement. Nurses tend to be broad and narrative when telephoning physicians.[10] They are taught early on in their education not to make direct cause-and-effect statements and not to make medical diagnoses, so they end up many times saying more than is necessary to explain a clinical picture. Although there are clearly times where bottom-line facts without expanded explanation can lead to poor decision making, as mentioned earlier, it is important for nurses to be specific, direct, and concise when providing feedback. State the problem clearly and provide objective data when able. Recall Carol's statement in the initial scenario with Dr. Smith. She provided lab values, vital sign data, and objective patient assessment data to support her concern.

Step 3

Step 3 of the assertive tool involves stating an alternative plan. Chances are if you are uncomfortable with a situation, you want something else to occur. That "something" is usually your proposed course of action. If a nurse contacts a physician regarding a patient's declining status and wants the patient to be clinically evaluated right away, then that needs to be stated as the desired plan. It may be a diagnostic test, transfer to a higher level of care, or prescribing a medication. Whatever it is, trust your assessment and judgment, believe in your ability to think critically, and know that it is not irreverent or pushy, or an attempt to practice medicine when a nurse asserts a well-thought-out position on behalf of a patient's safety. Nurses should avoid a paradigm that says only the physician has graduated from medical school, so therefore only he or she can steer medical decisions. Once a plan of action is suggested, agreement on whether that plan will be followed must be reached.

Step 4

Step 4 requires posing a question. Asking a question forces the receiver to respond. Stating concerns and proposing a plan go a long way in facilitating effective communication; however, the proposed receiver of that information is not obligated via normal discourse to respond to statements. The receiver is however socially obligated, or at the very least pressured, to respond to a direct question. The sender can still be ignored, but this moves into the realm of extreme rudeness if there is a refusal to answer a direct question. Pilots are taught that if someone fails to answer a question in the cockpit, the question should be asked again. If there is still no response, one must consider that the receiver may be incapacitated, which requires prompt investigation. In the cockpit, effective teams acknowledge all communications. For nurses, using the interrogative to secure agreement on a course of action when talking to any team leader, nurse, or physician must be done to complete an effective assertive statement.

There are those of us who are naturally assertive, those of us who can make our concerns and positions known without invoking the use of a tool or acronym. But many professionals are not naturally assertive and need help in advocating or disagreeing with a course of action in a dynamic situation. In fact, even the most assertive individuals can fall prey to hinting and hoping, or worse yet silence, in the face of hierarchy, intimidation, or emergent situations. The four-step tool can help; although it may be cumbersome at first and things may not come out perfectly when said aloud, it can be very effective if followed.

Let's go back to that cockpit on that snowy day in December to highlight an additional point about the four-step assertive statement. I mentioned the trigger or red flag that caused me to employ the assertive communication tool and, in a sense, snap into action. It is important to recognize those triggers and act on them. I also mentioned that the captain in this scenario, Tom, yelled expletives in my direction and did not receive my information in a respectful manner. His hard application of the brakes was entirely inappropriate for the passengers. While I did not appreciate this behavior, I did not address it in the heat of the moment. My only concern was safety, and Tom, although it wasn't pretty, did address that issue. It is important to avoid the trap of making things personal and getting wrapped up in a heated debate or argument. Handle the safety issues when things are dynamic. Deal with personal issues later when the situation is static, or stable. It is also important to remember that followership calls for assertiveness, not aggressive behavior. Followers must practice inquiry (question everything in their thoughts and speak when necessary) and advocacy (state openly a desired course of action, even if it is contrary to what the team leader or group is thinking). It is easy to see that if these two elements are carried out in a threatening, competitive, or overly aggressive manner, the value of the one's input can be diminished and everyone on the team is immediately placed on the defensive. You can say anything to anyone in the interest of safety, regardless of rank or title, provided rude or disrespectful dialogue is removed from the equation.

Escalation: Time to Up the Ante

As a follower, residing in the upper right quadrant of Kelly's model (See Figure 6.1) may not always be enough, especially when team leaders are not listening or are engaged. The 3Ws and the four-step assertive statement provide nurses with tools to ensure safe and desirable outcomes for patients. These tools should be used in an escalating fashion. First, use the 3Ws to offer feedback that is specific, direct, and concise. If that approach does not work, escalate to the four-step tool. If this is not successful in gaining resolution, then it is time to up the ante even further. At this point, you then use the chain of command. This could mean calling an attending physician, nursing supervisor, or charge nurse. Whoever that individual or point of contact may be, the chain of command is always an option to consider when all else fails. Consider the following true case, taken from the AHRQ Morbidity and Mortality Rounds (*www.webmm.ahrq.gov*):

A surgical resident is planning orthopedic surgery on an elderly gentleman. A cardiologist's evaluation has identified a history of aortic stenosis and strongly recommends that the surgery not be done. Even with spinal anesthesia, aortic stenosis increases the risk of hypotension and hypoperfusion of the coronary arteries resulting in sudden death. The resident comes to the floor and informs the nurse that the patient is scheduled for surgery at 7 p.m. that evening. The nurse attempts to provide the appropriate information to the surgical resident, but he doesn't listen, telling the nurse that they will not be doing general anesthesia, so there is nothing to worry about. After the resident leaves the unit, the nurse calls the facility's chief medical officer (CMO) and explains the situation. He quickly intervenes. The CMO immediately finds the resident, reviews the cardiologist's evaluation, and the case is cancelled.

This was a bold step on the part of the nurse and demonstrates the value of effective followership. Let's go back to the cockpit as there is yet another option to consider when escalating assertiveness.

On a snowy January day in 1982, Air Florida Flight 90 began its takeoff roll from what was then Washington National Airport in DC. As the aircraft slowly accelerated down the runway, the first officer became concerned with information he was seeing on cockpit instruments that indicated engine thrust. Cross-checking these indications, he was soon convinced that something was not right. He wasted no time and immediately raised the issue with the captain. In fact, he did so at least four times, at one point voicing his concern in the form of a question. The captain dismissed it. The first officer, although engaged and critically thinking, suddenly backed off; persuading himself that maybe he was not really seeing an abnormality after all. The aircraft lifted off but struggled to stay aloft. Seconds later, Flight

90 crashed onto the 14th Street Bridge, killing five people in their cars as they sat in traffic. The jet continued forward, impacted the frigid waters of the Potomac River, quickly disappearing beneath the ice. Only four passengers and a flight attendant survived after several dramatic rescue efforts.

On postcrash analysis of the cockpit voice recorder, or black box, listeners can hear what is called the "stick shaker" vibrating the pilot's control column, indicating to the crew that the wing of the aircraft was entering an aerodynamic stall and losing lift. The first officer was correct: something was drastically wrong. An engine probe had iced over and was sending erroneous information to the cockpit. The crew thought they were taking off with 100% thrust when in reality they had only applied about 70% of available takeoff thrust. This, coupled with a layer of ice and snow on the wings, proved to be a deadly combination. The purpose here is not to second-guess or criticize this copilot. He was an accomplished airman and part of an industry culture just beginning to expose itself to the benefits of CRM. That said, what else could the first officer have done in this case? The answer lies in one word: Action. This was a time-critical situation; as the aircraft gained speed and consumed available runway, the point of no return was rapidly approaching. Perhaps he could have attempted a more structured assertive statement, but when it became clear that the captain was not listening, the decision to grab the thrust levers, yank them to idle, apply the brakes, and abort the takeoff became a real option. Survival transcends obedience.

As nurses escalate their assertiveness to resolve clinical situations, they must understand that the **option to act must be considered**. Indeed, it is a bold step, but if a patient's life hangs in the balance, and time is short, action is always an option. What is the proper analogy within the nursing domain for a copilot grabbing the thrust levers in a jet aircraft and aborting a takeoff? Perhaps it is gently grabbing someone's arm to prevent administering a medication, or maybe it's calling a code or stopping an infusion pump. There are many possibilities here, but remember the central point: Effective followers consider taking action when situations are critical and time is running out.

Soaring to Success

Let's Put It All Together

Figure 6.2 is an effective followership algorithm that nurses can use to preserve operational safety in clinical situations. It encompasses all the tools discussed in this chapter.

Case study and exercise

The following narrative below was taken from the AHRQ Morbidity and Mortality Rounds (*www.webmm.ahrq.gov*). Read the following case and answer the questions below.

A 55-year-old obese woman with a history of hypertension and severe obstructive sleep apnea requiring continuous positive airway pressure (CPAP) is placed on morphine

FIGURE
6.2

Effective Followership Algorithm

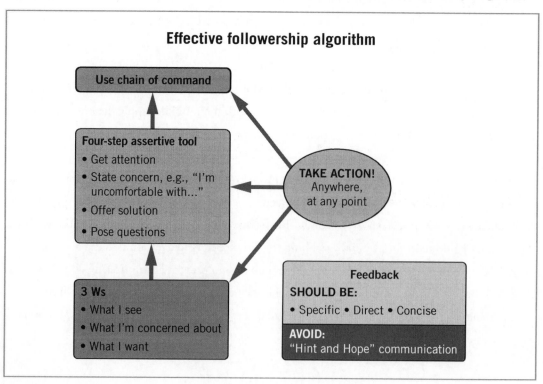

PCA pump for pain control following cholecystectomy. At approximately 1:00 a.m., five hours after starting the morphine, the patient's respiratory rate decreased to 7 (while on CPAP). Physical examination revealed an oxygen saturation level of 98%, normal blood pressure, heart rate of 50, and pinpoint pupils. The patient was noted to be lethargic, opening her eyes and mumbling incoherently in response to vigorous shaking but quickly falling asleep when the stimulus ceased. Concerned, the RN called the attending physician. The physician seemed annoyed by the call, barking, "What would you expect when you wake up a patient in the middle of the night from deep sleep—an excellent level of consciousness? Naturally, she would be drowsy!" He followed with, "Wake me up only on life and death issues!"

1. How would you initially conduct this phone call to provide specific, direct, and concise information? Use the **3Ws** as a guide.

2. After you receive the physician's response, you will need to escalate your level of assertiveness. Use the **four-step communication tool** to formulate your response.

Conclusion

In one sense, much of the discussion about followership and assertive communication seems simple. It's not rocket science. All that is required is to state what is wrong. How hard could that be?

It may not be rocket science, but effective communication can be difficult, even at the most rudimentary level, and does not occur with consistency. The Joint Commission cites communication as a root cause in almost 70% of all sentinel events.[18, 19] Nurses agree with this assessment. In 2006, the journal *Nursing* surveyed just under 5,000 nurses on patient safety topics. According to the survey, when presented with the following statement: Errors happen because of: 1) human failures, 2) system failures, or 3) communication failures, communication failures scored highest.

Soaring to Success

Recently I facilitated a seminar that taught CRM concepts to undergraduate nursing students. Of the topics covered, a good portion of the day was spent discussing followership and assertive communication. The students were given a scenario much like the case study of the oversedated woman. They were then asked to put together a four-step assertive statement to secure the appropriate outcome for their patient. This was an enlightening experience. Many students appeared self-conscious and awkward when using a tool to guide their communication. One particular student thought it was "stupid" to rehearse something that was so easy and simple. Others developed the statement relatively well, but spoke with a complete lack of confidence and emphasis. Not all had problems; some got the message and did quite well.

I have had similar experiences with seasoned nurses. Some were timid and had great difficulty utilizing formalized communication despite proclaiming themselves as "normally assertive" on the unit, while a few spoke forcefully but had trouble keeping it short and sweet. Others nurses assumed a defensive posture and sounded contentious and argumentative; some spoke with a complete lack of authority.

Although many experienced nurse clinicians do well putting a relevant assertive statement together, I continue to be struck by how difficult this can be for a group of professionals who shoulder so much responsibility. This underscores the need to expose nurses to CRM training often and early, as students and throughout their professional lives. Nurse leaders would be wise to champion such training. Communicating concisely and with specificity, routinely practicing inquiry and advocacy, using standardized tools to organize thoughts into assertive statements and action will assist nurses in their endeavor to keep patients safe.

References

1. Musson, D.M., G.M. Sandal, and R.L. Helmreich. Personality characteristics and trait clusters in final stage astronaut selection. *Aviation, Space, and Environmental Medicine. 2004; 75*:342–9. 2004; 76: p. 342–9.

2. Kelley, R. *The power of followership.* 1992, New York: Doubleday.

3. Kelley, R.E. In praise of followers. *Harvard Business Review, 1988,* 66(6): p. 142–148.

4. Powell, W. Trust based forms of governance, 293. In *Trust in Organizations,* R.M. Kramer, and T.R. Tyler, eds. 1996, Thousand Oaks, CA: Sage.

5. Tyler, T.R., and P. Degoey. Trust in Organizational Authorities, 332. In *Trust in Organizations,* R.M. Kramer, and T.R. Tyler, eds. 1996, Thousand Oaks, CA: Sage.

6. Tyler, T.R., and P. Degoey. Trust in Organizational Authorities, 343. In *Trust in Organizations,* R.M. Kramer, and T.R. Tyler, eds. 1996, Thousand Oaks, CA: Sage.

7. Sexton, J.B., E.J. Thomas, and R.L. Helmreich. Error, stress, and teamwork in medicine and aviation: cross sectional surveys. *British Medical Journal 2000; 320*: p. 745–749.

8. Powell, S., and R. Hill. My co-pilot is a nurse-using crew resource management in the OR. *AORN Journal* 2006, 83(1): 179–198.

9. Leonard, M., S. Graham, and D. Bonacum. The human factor: the critical importance of effective teamwork and communication in providing safe care. *Quality and Safety in Health Care* 2004, 13(suppl 1): i85–i90.

10. Leonard, M., S. Graham, and D. Bonacum. The human factor: the critical importance of effective teamwork and communication in providing safe care. *Quality and Safety in Health Care* 2004, 13(Supplement 1): i85–i90.

11. Neily, J., P. Mills, N. Eldridge, et al. Incorrect surgical procedures within and outside of the operating room. *Archives of Surgery* 2009, 144(11): 1028–1034.

12. Winters, D.D., A.P. Gurses, H. Lehmann, et al. Clinical review: Checklists - translating evidence into practice. *Critical Care* 2009, 13(6).

13. Sutcliffe, K.M., E. Lewton, and M.M. Rosenthal. Communication failures: an insidious contributor to medical mishaps. *Academic Medicine 2004; 79*: p. 186–194.

14. Lingard, L., S. Espin, S. Whyte, et al. Communication failures in the operating room: An observational classification of recurrent types and effects. *Quality and Safety in Health Care* 2004, 13: p. 330–334.

15. Schein, E.H. *Organizational Culture and Leadership,* 3rd ed, chapter 5. San Francisco: Jossey-Bass.

16. McFerran, S., J. Nunes, D. Pucci. Perinatal patient safety project: A multicenter approach to improve performance reliability at Kaiser Permanente. *Journal of Perinatal and Neonatal Nursing* 2005, 19(1): p. 37–45.

17. Uhlig, P.N., et al. Reconfiguring clinical teamwork for safety and effectiveness. *Focus on Patient Safety* 2002, 5(3): p. 1–2.

18. The Joint Commission. Preventing infant death and injury during delivery. *Sentinel Event Alert, 30.* 2004 [cited 2/21/2010]; Available from: *www.jointcommission.org/sentinel_event_alert_issue_30_preventing_ infant_death_and_injury_during_delivery/.*

19. The Joint Commission. *The Joint Commission Guide to Improving Staff Communication.* 2005, Oakbrook Terrace, IL: Joint Commission Resources.

CHAPTER 7

Situational Awareness: Making Clinical Decisions in the Nursing Environment

LEARNING OBJECTIVES

After reading this chapter, the participant will be able to:

- Identify the dangers posed by low situational awareness

- Discuss how the nursing environment makes situational awareness difficult

- List strategies that nurses can use to increase situational awareness

In Chapter 2, we discussed that to simplify things, crew resource management (CRM) can be thought of as having two main parts. So far, we have looked at the first: the interpersonal behaviors required to ensure that team communication truly supports higher levels of safety. Now, let's examine another aspect of CRM that is just as critical to team effectiveness: situational awareness (SA).

The term situational awareness is thrown around a lot in healthcare—especially when discussing errors and adverse events—but what does it really mean and why is it important? A good starting point is to first explore a formal definition of the term. Dr. Mica Endsley, a pioneer and world leader in the study and application of SA in advanced systems, offers the following definition: SA is defined as the perception of the elements within a volume of time and space, the comprehension of their meaning, and the projection of their status in the near future.[1, 2]

If you think about it, it's a very simple and straightforward explanation. First, individuals perceive things around them; then they give those "things" meaning based largely on the context of their circumstances. From here, they develop some idea of what might occur in the immediate or very near future.

SA is often described in terms of being either high, which is desirable, or low, which is not desirable. Pilots will often discuss their low SA when analyzing performance that is less than optimal. Low SA increases the chance for poor outcomes and adverse events in any operational setting. ◆

◆ Sidebar 7.1

Defining and measuring SA

There are more than 30 definitions and 20 methods of measuring SA, and most use some form of Endsley's definition as a basis.[3] Dominquez synthesized 15 SA definitions and then defined SA as an individual's "continuous extraction of environmental information, and integration of this information with previous knowledge to form a coherent mental picture, and the use of that picture in directing future perception and anticipating future events".[4]

Although there is no empirical evidence that directly validates these various models of SA, the main incongruence between the definitions lies in the reference to SA as either a process of gaining awareness (this is Endsley's point), or as the product of gaining awareness through a perceptual cycle. Some combine the two to initiate activity in a continuous sampling of the environment and updated understanding and prediction of the future state.[3, 5]

Simply put, SA is the term given to an operators' dynamic understanding of what is going on and what might be happening next.[6]

The Premise

I have had the opportunity to experience both the airline cockpit and the nursing unit from an operational perspective, which is why I can make the following statement: **It is exponentially more difficult for a nurse to maintain adequate levels of SA then it is for a pilot**. Here is why I make this assertion: For one thing, the cockpit is a controlled environment. There are two pilots in a relatively isolated area, operating one flight with a single well-defined mission, flying an aircraft that responds predictably 99% of the time. This is not the case on a nursing unit. Nurses have not one, but multiple patients, all of whom represent an independent entity for whom they must process information and make decisions. Patients are not as predictable as airplanes. Give the same medication to two patients, and you can get two completely different outcomes. Most significantly, unlike the cockpit, the nursing unit is loaded with interruptions, distractions, and human factor traps that greatly strain our limited cognitive resources.

I am not suggesting that developing and maintaining SA in the cockpit isn't a challenge, or that aviators cannot find themselves in some pretty dicey situations, but I am saying nurses have a more difficult operational environment, often with less cultural support.

Levels

To understand SA as a concept, let's look at how Endsley breaks it down into three levels. We can apply those levels to a clinical scenario.

Level 1

Level 1 SA is perception. This means that something reaches your senses; you smell it, feel it, hear it, taste it, or see it. Level 1 SA means that something has captured your attention, but that is all. For example, after assessing a patient, you detect that he has low blood pressure, tachycardia, low O_2 saturation, decreased urine output, changes in mental status, and is mildly febrile. You further recognize that the patient has a central line, which has been in place for about two weeks. Every one of these things has captured your attention; you are aware that each of these individual realities exists, but no further processing occurs. With Level 1 SA, individual elements reach your senses, but it stops there.

Level 2

With Level 2 SA, you go beyond simply being aware and attach meaning to those things that have captured your attention. You take the individual elements, put them together in some kind of order, and relate them to each other; this allows you to see things in a broader context. Put another way, rather than focus on individual trees, you begin to see a patch of woods, perhaps even a forest. When you look at our patient example, each element or piece of data (low blood pressure, tachycardia, altered mental status, etc.) by itself means nothing, but when you start putting the pieces of information together, a bigger picture begins to form. In fact, with appropriate Level 2 SA, it can be said that you are seeing the big-picture view, and it is from this view that we derive the significance of individual pieces of information and comprehend the overall meaning of a situation. Things start to make sense, and we are able to categorize and define scenarios. For this particular patient, when we put it all together, our big picture view says sepsis.

Level 3

At Level 3, we take our big-picture understanding of the situation and make projections about what may or may not happen in the immediate or near future. In the case of our patient—with the big picture that we have comprehended as sepsis—we start thinking ahead and can visualize outcomes. One highly probable outcome is that this patient will continue to decline, develop septic shock, and ultimately die from inadequate perfusion and subsequent organ failure. You know that the patient needs blood cultures, potent antibiotics, blood pressure support in the form of IV fluids and vasopressors, and monitoring to begin the process of sepsis resuscitation and management.[7] Based on this projection, you make decisions and perform actions such as calling the physician or the rapid response team, if available, to effect an immediate transfer to a higher level of care.

The key point here is that the products or endpoints of moving through these levels are decisions. It therefore makes sense to say that SA is the precursor to all decision making. Any decision you make as a nurse in the clinical area is only as good as the quality of SA that you possess at the time the decision is made. For example, if we do not perceive a very important piece of information because it fails to capture our attention, our decisions and actions will be flawed. If we perceive all relevant information but do not properly piece things together when forming the big picture, our decision and actions will be flawed. If we move through Levels 1 and 2 just fine, but fail to project how this will impact a patient's immediate future, our decisions and actions will be flawed. As nurses, we certainly do not set out to make poor decisions, so when we discuss SA, we must also explore not only the conditions in our operational environment that threaten SA, but also the limitations of our cognitive resources. The discussion of environmental threats and cognitive limits has great relevance in any setting, but none greater than the unique environment that is the nursing unit. First, we will explore threats and limitations, and then we'll look at strategies to manage them in the clinical environment.

Threats and Limitations

We only have so much attention to go around

SA is highly dependent on human attention. As we discussed, a starting point in developing SA and making decisions is simply being aware of something in the environment; a piece of information first has to capture our attention. This is problematic in that attention is a limited resource; we only have so much of it to go around. Suppose I am talking to a patient in the hallway on the unit. The patient is relaying a very important concern to me, and

I'm listening intently. The patient has my attention. Suddenly, I hear someone call my name and I turn my head in that direction to see a physician approaching with a question about a recently ordered medication. Now my attention is refocused for a moment, divided between the patient and the physician. As all of this is happening, I fail to see an elderly patient with dementia wandering out of an adjacent room and down the hall. Moments later, he falls and breaks a hip. ◆

◆ Sidebar 7.2
Divided attention and automacity

Complex operating environments invariably contain multiple goals that can all be active at the same time.[8] When an individual is performing several tasks at once, attention is divided among those tasks, which all have to be coordinated to prevent chaos.[9]

When performing these tasks, there will also be interruptions, which are those discrete events that must be addressed briefly. There will also be distraction by ongoing conditions.[10] These distractions and interruptions strain a person's cognitive resources and can produce a "looking without seeing" state for the operator.

Complex operating environments also lead to automacity, which is the term for directing one's gaze to a gauge or instrument and reading the expected or normal value rather than the indicated value.[10] We often "see" what we expect to see.

When I think about human attention, I envision a bucket. When the bucket gets full, we cannot pay attention to anything more. In order to add additional information to the bucket, we must pull our attention away from something else to make room, otherwise the bucket overflows. Nursing units have multiple sources of stimuli that relentlessly compete for our limited attention. This creates increased risk for patients and is a source of great stress and dissatisfaction for nurses at the point of care. As we will discuss in the next chapter, the risk is even more profound when our attentional resources are taxed during the performance of critical, safety-sensitive tasks. All too often there is simply too much coming at us, our attention buckets overflow, and we fail to pick up salient clinical information. Yet, as a professional group we tend to discount such human factor limitations and internalize poor patient outcomes, erroneously attributing clinical error and misadventure to individual failures.[11, 12] Knowing and accepting that attention is critical to the development of a nurse's SA, but also a limited resource, is the first step in developing strategies and countermeasures to reduce attention overload, thus giving nurses an opportunity to make sound clinical decisions.

Attentional narrowing

On a December night in 1972, Eastern Airlines Flight 401 approached Miami International Airport for landing.[13] The crew lowered the landing gear and quickly discovered that a problem existed. In the cockpit, when all three of the landing gear are down and locked in position, three green lights illuminate. On this night, only two lights illuminated so the crew knew it had a dilemma. Was it truly a mechanical failure or was it simply a burned-out lightbulb in the landing gear indicator? Flight 401 discontinued its approach and was instructed to maintain 2,000 ft. as they flew in the vicinity of the airport trying to diagnose and fix the problem. As things unfolded, all members of the crew became deeply involved in trying to analyze and remedy the situation before them. Unfortunately, as they did so the autopilot, which maintains altitude, was inadvertently disengaged and the aircraft entered a shallow and imperceptible descent, which the crew did not notice. At one point, a chime sounded, indicating that the aircraft had descended below its assigned altitude—but no one heard it.

It was a moonless night over the Florida Everglades, and as the aircraft slowly descended in the darkness, everyone in the cockpit continued focusing on the difficulty with the landing gear, unaware that the aircraft and all its occupants were in imminent danger. Seven seconds before impact, the first officer suddenly realized that they were no longer at 2,000 ft. and said, "We did something to the altitude" and "We're still at 2,000, right?" The captain replied by saying, "Hey, what's happening here?" Three seconds later, the sound of impact is heard as the aircraft crashed into the Everglades; there were ultimately 103 fatalities.

This type of accident is a phenomenon called controlled flight into terrain (CFIT). CFIT occurs when the crew loses SA and allows the aircraft to hit terrain in a normal flight attitude, not diving or descending out of control. The crew experienced "attentional narrowing." All of their attention resources were focused on the problem, so much so that they failed to monitor the altitude of the aircraft. The flight crew's final words are telling. When they finally began to realize that something was wrong with the altitude, their statements "We're still at 2,000, right?" and "Hey, what's happening here?" indicate that at that moment their SA was so profoundly low, they had difficulty accepting and processing the reality facing them. In those final seconds, no pilot made definitive thrust or flight control inputs in an attempt to alter the outcome; their big picture had become so small, they were in effect along for the ride. This is not an indictment of any individual member of the flight crew. On the contrary, attentional narrowing is a vulnerability that comes with being human. When human beings are under great stress, deeply involved in managing and resolving an abnormality or emergency, there is a natural tendency to focus, even fixate, on dominant information at the expense of peripheral factors. Many times these peripheral factors can be lethal in high-risk operations.

Just like the flight crew in the previous example, nurses experience highly stressful operational periods when patient abnormalities and emergencies must be effectively managed. They, too, are at risk for the pronounced reductions in SA, loss of peripheral information, and suboptimal decision making resulting from attentional narrowing. Consider the following example.

A nurse is caring for a patient experiencing abdominal pain and distention several days after hip replacement surgery. Because the patient has been receiving a full complement of IV and oral narcotics for postoperative analgesia, and has not had flatus or a bowel movement since before surgery, the nurse and resident physician

Soaring to Success

focus on reduced bowel function secondary to surgery as the cause of the problem. The patient is encouraged to ambulate and suppositories are given, but the pain continues. Enemas are ordered and administered with no relief. The patient's family grows increasingly upset as the pain worsens and demands that something be done to make their loved one comfortable. There are other clinical signs present such as low grade fever, mild nausea, and changes in routine laboratory tests collected earlier in the day, but they are subtle and attracting much less attention than the patient's discomfort. Several hours have gone by and now the patient's condition turns markedly worse. It is then correctly determined that the bowel has perforated postoperatively. The patient is brought to surgery for exploration and repair, but dies shortly thereafter from severe peritonitis.

As was the case with the Eastern Airlines crew, not attending to peripheral or less salient information lying outside the central focus of attention can be lethal. Rather than view the patient's pain among the backdrop of other clinical indicators to form a broader picture of the situation (higher degree of SA), the team focuses on the most demanding piece of information, placing great emphasis on immediate pain relief. For the patient, precious time is lost during this period of attentional narrowing.

Working memory

Whereas Level 1 SA is closely linked with human attention, other levels of SA are highly dependent on the working memory (also called short-term memory). After information in the clinical environment captures our attention, we place it in the working memory for processing. What's happening now? What does all this information mean? (Level 2 SA comprehension) Now that I have determined what's happening, what can I expect (Level 3 SA, projection), and what should I do about it? (decisions). One could say that the working memory is the psychological venue in which critical thinking takes place; it's where the action is. It is the thinking, processing, and sense making we accomplish in real time.

Distinguished psychologist James Reason explains that the working memory is closely linked to what he calls the "conscious workspace, the experiential here and now".[14] To describe the conscious workspace, he asks you to picture yourself on a bank watching a stream go by. The stream curves around a sharp bend as it moves toward you, and again curves around another bend as it moves away. You can't see upstream or downstream; all you can see is the part that swiftly passes in front of you. The clinical information you process on the unit in real time is the part of the stream that you can see. Reason's metaphor is an excellent way to describe the "here and now" aspect associated with working memory. Formally, working memory can be defined as the limited number of ideas sounds or images that we are able to maintain and manipulate mentally at any point in time.[15] The key word in this definition is "limited."

Working memory capacity

Just like the attention resource, working memory is a cognitive resource with finite capacity, like a bucket. We can maintain about five to seven items, or chunks, of information in the working memory at any one time, after which the bucket overflows, and the information is not recalled. For nurses this is significant because the information they place in their working memories is patient assessment data that ultimately drive clinical decisions. When a nurse assesses a patient in any setting, the working memory receives multiple bits of information. Nursing units are dynamic places, things can happen fast, so we often depend on our working memory capacity to maintain information. It is not always possible to write things down or place them in a computer charting database right away.

Envision a nurse rounding on a patient at the start of a shift. Information gathered during the assessment of the patient is:

- The heparin infusion is on hold pending lab results per hospital protocol so the latest Partial Thromboplastin Time (PTT) will need to be checked

- The IV site is red and painful and needs to be restarted

- Patient started a new IV antibiotic today

- Blood pressure is elevated

- The CT scan of the chest that was ordered for today should have been done already but has not yet occurred; needs to be followed up on

- Patient has a rash on his chest and arm

- The patient's lower right extremity is still markedly swollen

- The patient is adhering to bed rest

There are eight independent items all gathered from this assessment, some that possibly relate to each other, some that are independent, and others that require action and follow-up in order of priority. Just with this one patient, we can see that the working memory bucket fills up fast. It's not hard to imagine the nurse several hours later realizing that he forgot to address the CT scan of the chest. The takeaway point here is the amount of information we can place and maintain in the working memory is limited. If capacity is exceeded, some information gets pushed out and is forgotten. ◆

◆ Sidebar 7.3

Limits of memory and chunking

One of the most frequently cited papers in psychology is "The magical number seven plus or minus two: Some limits on our capacity for processing information" by George Miller.[16] In his discussion of memory span, Miller found the short-term memory span of young adults is approximately seven items. The idea of a "magical" number has inspired much theorizing regarding the capacity limits of human cognition. Later research on short-term memory found that memory span is not constant in terms of what is recalled (e.g., numbers, letters, single syllable words, multi-syllable words) or how the information is organized (i.e., random words or words organized into a sentence).[17]

This has led to a deeper understanding of Miller's work that implies placing information within a context or "chunks" can extend the reach of memory. Chunking refers to the strategy of combining separate items of cognition into a single mental unit that allows us to deal with many items as though they were one.[18] For example, when recalling a 10-digit phone number, such as 6973487342, we might break this into 69-73, 48-73, and 42. In this manner we are remembering five groups of numbers and not 10 separate digits.[19]

We can use chunking in the case we just discussed. For example, the nurse has eight pieces of data to remember. Some of them are related, so they are easily chunked together to aid retention. In this situation, the nurse groups the three related actions together—check lab for IV heparin, new IV antibiotic started, needs new IV started—and can recall all of them by simply recalling the term "IV."

Another limit of the working memory is time. Research indicates that items we place in the working memory will begin to decay in as little as 20 seconds unless that information is used and acted on. Other sources place the point at seven seconds for three chunks and 70 seconds for one chunk.[15, 20] Pilots often receive navigational clearances with multiple items from air traffic control that must first be read back and then carried out.

A controller may instruct a pilot to "Turn left to a heading of 270 degrees, descend and maintain 5,000 feet, and reduce speed to 180 knots." If the pilot has to delay the readback of the instructions for any reason, unless it is written down, the information begins to decay and becomes difficult to recall correctly.

Nurses are visible on multibed med–surg units. They come in contact with multiple people within a given time frame and are often the recipient of unsolicited verbal information at inopportune times from patients, physicians, and other staff. For example, while quickly leaving the unit to respond to an emergency, a physician stops a nurse in the hall and says; "With Mr. Jones in 356, we need to discontinue the Foley catheter, change the IV to a saline lock, discontinue his IV pain medications, and get a CBC in the a.m."

The nurse places these items in her working memory and holds on to this information until it can be written, typed, or acted upon, thus unloading her memory. Chances are there will be either delays or interruptions before having the opportunity to do so; at which point significant information decay occurs, causing some of the items to be forgotten.

The Load on Working Memory

The working memory is the place where real-time information processing occurs, which is crucial to the development of higher degrees of SA. Let's briefly discuss a simplified version of this information processing, and the load that is placed on working memory in a given clinical situation.

In Figure 7.1, we see three buckets representing our cognitive resources, or as I like to say, the mental machinery involved in the production of SA. The attention bucket on the left represents the resource that receives patient information from the environment. As mentioned earlier, the working memory bucket represents the place where we store and analyze the information in the here and now so we can make sense of what is happening. The long-term memory bucket represents all the information that we have learned and stored over time, either in the classroom, in training, or real-life experiences.

FIGURE
7.1

The Cognitive Resource of Situational Awareness

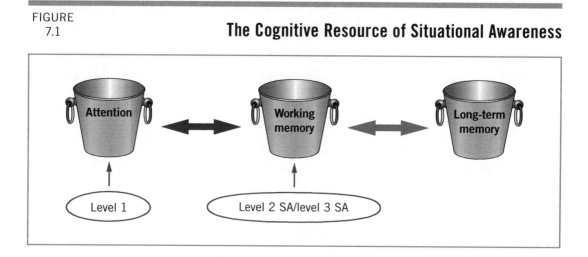

Recall the patient we discussed at the start of the chapter who exhibited multiple clinical signs that we identified as sepsis. How did we know this? We knew it because we have learned the pattern of sepsis. We've read case studies in texts and journals, learned about it in class, seen it before on the unit, and have learned to recognize it.

All of this information is stored in the long-term memory. So, when real time clinical data enter our working memory (does not decay or is not lost because memory capacity is exceeded), we compare what we are seeing with models, rules, schematics, and past experiences that reside in our long-term memory. This mental exchange, represented by the light gray two-way arrow in Figure 7.1, is how we understand, define, and comprehend a situation, allowing us to achieve Level 2 SA.

We have also learned what to do once we recognize sepsis, what clinical progression to expect, and the most appropriate course of action to take. This is the knowledge that gives us the predictions and projections characteristic of Level 3 SA, where we are again accessing mental models constructed and filed in our long-term memory. ◆

> ◆ Sidebar 7.4
> ## Building mental models on experience
>
> One of the key assumptions of Endsley's three-level model is that mental models play a critical role in the development and maintenance of SA. According to Endsley, environmental inputs are mapped to preexisting mental models that have been formed though previous training and experience, which in turn allow for attention to be directed to critical elements, an understanding of meaning developed, and a prediction of future states.[3]
>
> This explains why people with better developed (and tested) mental models can develop higher levels of SA than a novice who lacks recognition-primed (pattern-matching) decision-making ability gained through experience.[21] For example, Klein notes that experienced researchers classify problems differently than novices. In healthcare scenarios, two practitioners may have the same SA levels but choose different courses of action based on their prior clinical experience.[21]

These mental models are based largely on our expertise, derived from the practical experience and know-how we have acquired over time. For example, a novice nurse may correctly comprehend that a patient is septic, but not possess the requisite experience to know that immediate action is required, whereas a more experienced nurse possesses a mental model that tells her to urgently seek a higher level of care for this patient with sepsis.

The dark gray arrow on Figure 7.1 depicts the two-way interface between the attention resource and working memory. As discussed, the attention resource provides information for processing in the working memory. However, once we develop an understanding of a clinical situation, we use that understanding to guide subsequent assessments of the patient. In other words, once we know what's going on (Level 2 SA), we then have a good idea of where we should be looking for additional information (Level 1 SA). In this sense, working memory aids attention, thus the two way arrow. Perception is not only dependent on the ability of something in the environment to capture our attention, it is also aided by our ability to consciously direct our attention in the right place to sample the most pertinent information.[15, 22] For example, if your comprehension of clinical assessment information leads you to the conclusion that a patient has an altered level of consciousness, you will then direct your attention to specific assessment items to acquire additional information: check for head injury from a fall; check blood glucose; check blood pressure, etc.

The main point of the discussion is to highlight the enormous load that can be imposed on the working memory as we process clinical information. The working memory receives disjointed raw data from the world, makes sense of the data by comparing them with things we already know, patterns we can recognize. It then guides further assessment by directing the attention resource to specific places in the world to capture additional information, and it plays a role in making predictions about future conditions, which form the basis for decisions and actions. Even as all of this is going on, the working memory is still actively acquiring new data while holding on to existing chunks of information.[22] Wow! This is a tall order in the friendliest of environmental conditions. Unfortunately, we know that nursing units can be anything but friendly to cognitive processing, and there are many forces that diminish not only the capacity of the working memory, but its effectiveness in developing higher levels of SA.

Attention and working memory are linked

Attention and working memory are both limited resources, and they draw upon each other.[2] Metaphorically speaking, if we are in situations that seriously challenge or overload working memory, the working memory bucket becomes full, overflowing into the attention bucket, thus reducing the number of things we can pay attention to. Case in point: If we place pilots in a simulator and give them a complex abnormality that requires concentration and the deep application of technical knowledge, they may become so involved in synthesizing information that they fail to hear an audible chime indicating an additional problem. The reverse is also true. Take those same pilots and give them a continuous series of abnormalities, one after the other, each with their associated aural, visual, and tactile warnings. Chances are much of their time will be spent struggling to simply perceive, rather than engage in the processing that comes with higher levels of SA. Their attention bucket overflows into that of the working memory, reducing the ability to make sense of things. It is not difficult to imagine similar analogies in the nursing domain.

Environment

At the start of this chapter, I made the assertion that it is exponentially harder for a nurse to maintain SA than it is for a pilot. I make this statement from experience and stand by it. This is mainly because nurses have not one, but multiple, patients for whom they must perceive, comprehend, project, make decisions, and perform actions. Complicating the issue of multiplicity is the nature of the practice environment existing on today's inpatient multibed nursing units which can be replete with noise, interruptions, intense production pressure, poor human factor design, and cultural dysfunction. As stated, pilots operate in a relatively isolated and controlled environment, whereas nurses do not. Although the environments may differ greatly between the unit and the cockpit, there are similarities to the baseline challenges both professional groups when it comes to SA.

The following lists some of the more prominent stressors and threats to SA that have been identified in the aviation environment:

- Mental load

- Task load

- Time pressure

Soaring to Success

- Distractions

- Emergencies

- Fatigue

- Automation

Is there a nurse alive who has ever practiced who can say he or she has not dealt with any or all of these threats? When considering the unique nature of a nurse's professional practice environment, we might emphasize additional impediments to the development of SA, such as:

- Culture

- Intimidation

- Poor standardization

- Poor communication

- Poor teamwork

Remember that even in the best of circumstances, our cognitive resources are limited. Add these environmental threats to the mix, and the capacities of attention and working memory are further reduced. In the cockpit, threats that are not managed properly can cause attentional narrowing, poor SA, errors, and possibly mishaps. Recall the Eastern Airlines CFIT example. In the nursing domain, an outcome strongly analogous to CFIT is failure to rescue, subtle changes in a patient's condition going undetected, ultimately resulting in death. We might also consider outcomes such as falls with injury, medication errors, and interventions carried out on the wrong patient as additional CFIT analogies.

Now that we have defined SA and discussed the limits of our cognitive resources and the environmental threats that reduce SA, let's look at strategies that can be used in the nursing practice environment to preserve and maintain higher levels of both individual and team SA.

Strategies and Countermeasures for the Maintenance of SA

Avoiding premature closure

As stated, nurses experience highly stressful operational periods when patient problems, abnormalities, and emergencies must be effectively managed. In such situations, stress induces a tendency to arrive at a decision and act on it without exploring all available information.[1, 2] This is called premature closure, and it serves to degrade SA. Notice I did not say all information, but all *available* information. It's not possible to know everything, but it is crucial to know what is available to us. Remember, decisions are dependent upon what we process in our working memory, and what we process is dependent on the totality of the information we acquire from the environment. To avoid premature closure, it is important to first recognize that you are in the midst of a time-constrained situation requiring management and decision making. Then, before you make a decision and act, use the 1-2-3 rule:

LEADERSHIP TIP	Here is an SA tip: Use the 1-2-3 rule to increase your SA. 1. Step back 2. Ask, "Are we missing something?" 3. Use your resources

Whether you are alone, or by a patient's bedside with other members of the patient care team, saying the 1-2-3 rule silently or aloud provides the needed pause to ensure that the team is not missing key items that could affect the clinical decision being made. It's not a bad idea to physically take a step or two backward to emphasize this momentary pause in the action. This assumes, of course, that immediate critical needs are addressed as necessary. For example, you would certainly maintain a patient's airway first before stepping back. In the cockpit when there is a problem or emergency, a checklist is consulted. At some point in the checklist, it directs the flight crew to either "land as soon as possible," which means land now, or "land as soon as practical," which means there is time to consider more options. Unless your patient is experiencing a land as soon as possible scenario (airway, breathing, and circulation), most likely there is time to seek and consider more information (land as soon as practical). Actually say out loud, "Are we missing something?" If you are alone, say it out loud to yourself. Often just saying this will allow you to notice something obvious that you initially overlooked. If nothing else, it forces you to slow down. The third step, "use your resources," taps into the very essence of CRM. The most important resource you have is your team. Get them involved. It may be another nurse but it may also be a pharmacist or respiratory therapist. Perhaps a housekeeper has information you are unaware of. Resources may also be a piece of technology or a computer database. In Chapter 4, we discussed that leaders who practice good CRM know their resources. The "1-2-3 rule" prompts you to utilize those resources to support SA in the management of clinical problems.

Earlier I mentioned Captain Chesley Sullenberger and would now like to return to that January day in 2009 when he successfully ditched a US Airways Airbus 320 in the Hudson River. When the crew was a few hundred feet above the water, basically committed to ditching the aircraft after repeated attempts to restart both engines, Sullenberger asks the first officer, "Do you have any ideas?" The first officer responds, "Actually not."[23] This is an incredible act, the manifestation of years immersed in a culture that teaches and values CRM. Even in the midst of enormous operational pressure, Captain Sullenberger has the presence of mind to step back, if even for a moment, and use his crew. What he is saying here is that before we put this thing in the water, is there something staring us in the face, something that we missed, or some suggestion you have that might change the outcome. Impressive!

The next time you find yourself in a situation where you are challenged to manage a clinical problem of uncertain etiology and outcome, remember the 1-2-3 rule.

Task load division to ensure attention distribution

CRM is about managing resources effectively, so it makes complete sense that when task load is high, as it is on most patient care units, the work should be strategically divided among the team. Dividing up the workload ensures two things: 1) Individuals are not placed at greater risk for low SA due to task saturation and depletion of the attention resource, and 2) everyone on the team is not focused on the same thing (attentional narrowing)

This is the premise from which I strongly advocate a team approach to nursing care. By this I specifically mean that more than one staff member is assigned to the care of a patient, and each staff member is responsible for different tasks. This, in my view, is preferable to primary nursing which, for the sake of this discussion, means a model of care where one licensed nurse carries out all aspects of a patient's care on the unit: custodial care, medications, care planning, treatments, assessments, and communicating with physician providers. Primary care has its merits and is appropriate in certain conditions, but one must consider the fact that on many medical–surgical units, nurse–patient ratios are simply not conducive to sustaining this type of model. Without getting into extended discussion about nurse staffing ratios, I will assert that when human resources are challenged within a primary care model, the natural limits of our cognitive resources are easily exceeded. The result is low SA and the potential for poor decisions, increasing the risk for poor patient outcomes. Dividing the task load can take many forms such as designating a specific nurse(s) to:

- Administer medications

- Admit patients

- Discharge patients

- Review orders, complete assessment, and communicate with physicians

- Accomplish all IV site, tubing, and dressing changes (often overlooked)

- Perform treatments

- Obtain scheduled blood glucose measurements and administer insulin products

As you will read in Chapter 8, a team approach is nothing new. However, arguing for such a model in the name of preserving our limited cognitive resources of attention and working memory to support SA may be novel in the nursing arena of ideas. It is important to note that preserving the SA of each individual nurse on the unit is a precursor to the development of heightened overall team SA.

Some argue that dividing up the workload creates silos, organizational slang describing a phenomenon in which a focus only on one's own job prevails at the expense of teamwork and communication. As you will see, this was a common complaint from the nurses involved in the team care delivery model discussed in Chapter 8. Nurses felt that while they were relieved of task pressure by designating a patient care nurse and a medication delivery

◆ Sidebar 7.5

Team SA

Up to this point, we have examined individual SA. We now shift to SA in terms of the complex socio-technical teams found in healthcare.

The increasing complexity of the healthcare environment has led to the increased use of teams to accomplish care.[3] Teams are defined as two or more people dealing with multiple information sources while interacting dynamically, independently, and adaptively with specific roles and a limited lifespan of membership to accomplish a shared or common goal.[24, 25] Teams have been shown to perform difficult and complex tasks better, have better performance under stress, have fewer errors, and have improved decision-making capability than individual operators.[25]

Team SA is more complex than individual SA because it is multi-dimensional; it comprises individual team member's SA as well as the shared SA between team members, and it also includes the combined SA of the entire team. Because collaboration between team members requires complex exchanges of information, largely accomplished through spoken language, linguistic communication is the keystone of team performance in this regard[26]. See Figure 7.2 for a team SA diagram.

FIGURE
7.2

Team SA

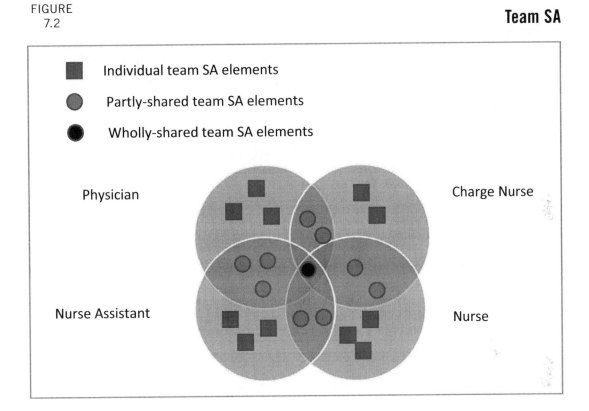

- ■ Individual team SA elements
- ● Partly-shared team SA elements
- ● Wholly-shared team SA elements

Physician

Charge Nurse

Nurse Assistant

Nurse

nurse, each did not have a complete picture of the patient because each individual was focused on his or her specific task, basically operating in silos. I would respond by saying that silos are not the problem, it's poor communication processes that are the problem. Task load division demands that a well-defined communication process be in place. Division of workload is a way of life in the cockpit, but this is supplemented with standardized callouts, checklists, and briefings to ensure effective communication. The same is true for us; if we divide up task load on the unit in support of SA, then we must supplement that model with standardized communication, briefings, and checklists. ◆

Bottom-line Behaviors

The Eastern Airlines CFIT crash in the everglades occurred in 1972, well before the advent of CRM. Today, crews that are well trained in CRM understand the concept of bottom-line safety behaviors. These are behaviors that must be accomplished at all costs no matter how chaotic things become. A bottom-line behavior in the cockpit is that someone must always fly the plane no matter what. If an aircraft is on fire, or it is depressurizing at high altitude, someone still has to fly the aircraft and monitor its flight path.

In other words, before the team begins managing an abnormality or emergency, bottom-line behaviors must first be attended to. The first thing a captain is trained to do when managing any problem on the flight deck, without fail, is ensure that some crew member has positive control of the aircraft at all times. So, in the case of the malfunctioning landing gear previously discussed, a captain trained in CRM would respond by saying the following to his copilot, "I will transfer control of the aircraft to you. I want you to maintain heading and altitude. I will run the landing gear failure checklist and talk to air traffic control. OK?" This is dividing up the task load to achieve bottom-line safety behaviors.

Nurses know what it feels like to be out there on the unit trying to complete routine tasks and manage the common and not-so-common elements of patient care while multiple patients are admitted, discharged, and recovered from surgery in a compressed time frame. That horrible feeling in the pit of your stomach, that little voice that says, "Things are happening with my patients that I'm not seeing" or "I haven't been in that patient's room in a long time and I don't know what I'm going find when I get there." These are indicators that chaos is replacing structure, and SA is running low.

It is in these situations that nurses should consciously refocus themselves on making sure that, if nothing else, at least bottom-line safety behaviors are addressed, because under great stress and task load, there may be a tendency to shed these behaviors in an effort to keep up. So, what are the bottom-line safety behaviors in nursing? What is the nursing equivalent to "fly the airplane"? The list may vary and it is not long, but my experience over the years when posing this question to groups of nurses is that two specific behaviors critical to patient safety consistently emerge:

- Assessment

- Patient identification

Assessment does not mean that a textbook head-to-toe physical assessment is completed. It does, however, mean that we at least lay eyes on the patient. We make sure they are physiologically stable and safe from harm or injury. Assessment bottom lines can be more specific as we move into different specialties. For example, if you practice on an oncology unit, a bottom-line assessment item may be verifying IV line patency and blood return before infusing a vesicant. Patient identification must precede all nursing actions, in all specialties, in every situation, including emergencies. You may think of additional bottom-line safety behaviors. For example, we might add hand washing to this list. The list should not be long as these are critical nursing actions that transcend all others.

As a clinician it is prudent to identify and revisit bottom-line safety behaviors, both individually and with your team. Talk about them in briefings, and post them on the unit in different places as a safety reminder. Remember, when we are pressured, falling behind and losing SA, we may overlook these simple but critical steps, yet without them, nothing else matters. In the cockpit, it is not uncommon to hear, "Let's be sure someone is flying the airplane." The analogy in our world is a charge nurse briefing the team saying, "OK, guys, let's be sure we assess the patient."

Remember: When things get chaotic, think bottom lines.

Recognizing and Responding to Clinical Red Flags

Clinical red flags are indicators in the environment that speak to us. They tell us that our SA may be low or at risk.[27, 28] When we recognize a red flag, the biggest thing to remember is not to press forward with decisions or actions until we investigate and resolve the issue. Red flags many times come to us by way of that little voice inside our head, a slow realization that something isn't quite right. ◆

> ◆ Sidebar 7.6
> ### Recognizing and organizing weak signals
>
> That little voice in our head is asking us to pay attention to what are at present only feelings, imprecise early indications, or weak signals that may be early signs that trouble lies ahead. A weak signal is a factor hardly perceptible at present, but that will constitute a huge factor in the future. Our normal tendency is to respond to a weak signal with a weak response because our energies and attention are needed elsewhere. But the little voice is asking that we connect the dots and organize the weak signals at our attentional periphery, incorporating them into a better picture of what is actually going on[29-31].

Listen to that voice; often it is the first step in regaining acceptable levels of SA. Once a clinical red flag is recognized, say it to yourself, and certainly say it aloud if you are among other members of the team. It is not a bad idea to include red flag recognition in unit briefings to emphasize the point that any member of the team can and should speak out when one is detected.

Once identified and spoken aloud, the next step is to resolve the red flag. Resolving the flag may require independent action if working alone, or require input from others if the situation involves a team working closely together in one place at the same point in time such as in a code, bedside procedure, or unit-based procedure requiring moderate sedation. A great tool/memory aid to assist us when recognizing and resolving a red flag is the 3Ws (What I see, What I am concerned about, What I want) discussed in Chapter 6. This not only encourages vocalizing concerns the moment they are known, but is in keeping with previous discussions about assertive communication in team settings. In any case, it is crucial to build a unit safety culture in which common red flags are defined and every member of the team is empowered to raise them.

The following sections list and explain common examples of clinical red flags.

Failed cross-check

If I were flying an airplane and one navigational instrument told me I was 150 miles east of Los Angeles, while another told me I was 150 miles south of Los Angeles, it would be best not to make any turns until I knew which one was telling me the truth. If independent sources of information that should agree do not, that's a failed cross-check. For example, you walk into a patient's room who has been hospitalized for several days with a cup full of medications. As you prepare to administer them, the patient says, "Wow, that's a lot of pills." You wouldn't expect this from a patient who routinely receives these medications. You recognize the situation as a red flag and discover that you inadvertently walked into the wrong room.

Failure to meet targets

An expected response after the initiation of a therapy or treatment does not occur as expected. For example, a patient is in respiratory distress and you receive an order for oxygen 100% via face mask. Fifteen minutes later the patient's O_2 saturation has not recovered and she is still short of breath. When we initiate any kind of therapy for a patient, we expect a clinical response within a defined time period. If that does not occur, it is a red flag and we may not be seeing the big picture. You step back and investigate to find that the respiratory therapist attached the face mask to the wall air adapter instead of the oxygen adapter.

Not addressing discrepancies

This occurs when we fail to act on elements in a clinical scenario that present incongruencies not normally expected. The discrepancies can be obvious, but often times are more subtle.

Soaring to Success

You report to the unit at the start of a shift and encounter a patient in the hall on a stretcher whom you admitted several days prior. The patient tells you that he is going for a CT scan with contrast. As they are wheeled off the unit, you remember that when you admitted them, they mentioned something about being allergic to contrast dye, but you aren't sure. You start to walk away and move onto something else, but you stop yourself, recognize the discrepancy, and call down to the CT suite and alert them to verify the patient's allergies.

Failure to delegate

Managing workload is central to practicing good CRM and required if we are to maintain higher levels of SA. Tasks that can be addressed by other available resources must be assigned as such. An example of a failure to delegate occurs when a nurse, while monitoring an unstable patient during the first few minutes of a blood transfusion, becomes involved in removing old linen from the bathroom, changing bed linen, and emptying an overflowing trash can. Or an RN who has his hands full managing a group of clinically challenging patients, struggles to admit a new patient and neglects to have an LPN complete part of the admission assessment for him. In both cases, SA is preserved when the lack of delegation is recognized as a red flag and then remedied.

Not following policy

This occurs when someone on the patient care team completes a process or action that is prohibited by policy or when someone fails to complete a process or action that is required by policy. Many times this red flag is a result of behavioral norms that, although deviant, are practiced by many. Often reasons for not following policy are: "I don't have enough time"; "The process is not realistic for the real-life clinical environment"; "I would like to be able to do that but there just isn't enough staff"; "I know that's what the policy says, but no one ever does that." A nurse working on a surgical unit initiates a heparin infusion on a patient without performing a check of the dosage at the bedside with another staff member. It's late in the shift and there is not another RN immediately available. She sets up the infusion knowing that when the nurse on the next shift arrives, she will verify the infusion on her rounds. If we ever hear that little voice in our head that says, "I know the policy says this but ...", you have just recognized a major red flag. Stop and fix it!

Confusion

In 1995, American Airlines 965 was on approach in mountainous terrain to the Alfonso Bonilla Aragon International Airport in Cali, Colombia. The crew became confused about their position while programming a navigational computer. At one point the copilot said aloud "Uh, where are we?" Three minutes later they crashed into a mountain. This is a classic CFIT accident due to loss of SA. The red flag presents as the ongoing discussion and confusion about the aircraft's position. The fact that the crew pressed onward in the presence of prolonged navigational uncertainty while descending in mountainous terrain is evidence that they did not recognize it. After a terrain warning sounded in the cockpit, the crew immediately regained the big picture and snapped into action, initiating an escape maneuver, but it was not successful. If we could rewrite this scenario, the feeling of confusion would be recognized, spoken aloud, and then acted on. Encountering clinical findings that do not make sense can leave any clinician with that nagging feeling of uncertainty and confusion. If you feel it, recognize it, speak it, and investigate.

Fixation

Spending too much time and directed attention on one clinical finding, problem, or aspect of a patient's care, or one patient within a group of patients, defines this red flag. For example, a nurse has a patient who needs parenteral antibiotics for severe cellulitis. The patient's physician emphasized to the nurse while rounding the critical importance of prompt antibiotic therapy. The patient is not able to have a peripherally inserted central catheter (PICC) placed right away; the nurse has tried several times over the last hour without success to establish IV access. She has not seen her other patients within that time frame, nor has she talked with the nursing assistant that is working with her.

Not communicating

Team members simply stop talking and sharing information with each other. This might occur for several reasons. When individuals become fatigued, one manifestation is that they stop interacting with the team. This flag can also occur when team leaders fail to share information that the rest of the team should know. The converse of this situation occurs when a subordinate team member fails to inform the team leader, as well as other team members, of important findings that may influence decision making. Not communicating may also occur when the communication loop is not actively closed; this happens when information is not "read back," or when information that lacks clarity is not questioned, allowing ambiguity to remain. For instance, when discussing a patient, an LPN receives instructions from the charge nurse to inform him if she encounters anything important in her assessment. The LPN wonders specifically what "important" means, but nods in agreement and moves on. Another example might occur when two nurses are caring for a patient who is not doing well. As they move in and out of the room performing tasks and collecting information, they fail to interact and/or discuss their findings with each other. In both cases, the chance for higher levels of SA is supported if a member of the team recognizes either the lack of verbal communication or lack of clarity in communication as a red flag.

FIGURE
7.3   **Red Flag Recognition Using the 3Ws**

The patient is suddenly tachypnic, anxious, and diaphoretic. Two RNs, an LPN, and a nursing assistant are at the patient's bedside. Vital signs are recorded and oxygen is applied. Blood pressure is lower than normal. Several minutes have gone by and the team seems stuck and cannot discern what is happening. The LPN says:

- **What I see:** "We're confused here and things are not getting better."

- **What I'm concerned about:** "I think we're missing something and we need to get some help."

- **What I want:** "Let's call the rapid response team."

Team Monitoring

Earlier I discussed the benefits of standardization. One of those benefits is that it allows us to predict the behavior of others on the team in the operational environment. If team members do not behave as expected, it must be investigated. People can become ill, momentarily incapacitated, or experience low SA, all of which create operational hazards. During an airline trip, one pilot will fly the aircraft and the other will assume nonflying-related duties.

In airline procedure manuals, all duties are clearly designated for each crew member. The pilot that physically flies the aircraft is called the PF, which stands for pilot flying. The pilot not flying the aircraft is designated as the PM, or pilot monitoring. This terminology is used for a reason. It emphasizes the monitoring function and responsibility of the crew member not flying the aircraft. If the PF fails to adhere to standard flight and crew communication profiles, the PM questions the PF. If there is no response, the PM must be prepared to take control of the situation. CRM dictates that each member of the crew monitors the behavior of the other, and if standards are not followed it must be promptly challenged.

Nursing units are not cockpits, but the same process of team monitoring should apply here as well. Some multibed nursing units are fortunate enough to have a "free" or "float" charge nurse, which in this discussion means a nurse who has a no direct patient care assignment (or a reduced direct patient care assignment) but who provides oversight and support in the completion of clinical activities for a shift. These nurses are extremely valuable as they serve as a resource to staff in troubleshooting clinical problems, assisting with tasks, and managing the flow of patients to and from the unit. The reality in professional nursing however is that the "free" charge nurse is considered a luxury, and often not supported in staffing plans. This is unfortunate because one of the most important functions this nurse can provide is team monitoring in support of SA and clinical decision making. I suggest changing the name of the "free" charge nurse to "Monitoring Charge Nurse" (MCN) to emphasize this point. Let's face it; right now as you read this, in hospital corridors across the country, there are nurses

Soaring to Success

standing in front of medication carts who are task saturated, fatigued, suffering the effects of depleted cognitive resources, with low SA, but no one will ever know. When we do become aware of this unfortunate predicament, it is often too late for the patient. Monitoring the status and behavior of others is required in a true safety culture. The purpose here is not to argue the business case for patient safety; this has been eloquently accomplished by others.[32, 33] Within that context, however, I will assert that building the MCN into staffing plans is a prudent use of resources in reducing the risk to hospitalized patients, not an expendable luxury.

Whether there is a MCN or not, nurses should buddy up and get into the habit of monitoring their teammates throughout the shift for signs that may indicate reduced SA. This goes beyond simply asking someone if they need help; this is monitoring professional behavior for adherence to standards. Nurses take pride in their expertise and expect a lot of themselves. Nurses also have a history of being harsh in judging their own performance, as well as the performance of peers,[34] especially those who have made errors in the past. For this reason being "watched" by others on the team may not be embraced with open arms. The culture must move past this punitive paradigm. ◆

Team monitoring is not judgmental, nor is it a competency evaluation. It is simply a logical safeguard in identifying and rescuing practitioners suffering from the effects of human factor limitations.

◆ Sidebar 7.7
Monitoring

In the complex, dynamic work environments of healthcare, no single individual can acquire the varied and often rapidly expanding information needed for success. It is necessary to shift analysis of cognition from the individual, such as is done in discussing critical thinking, to the entire cognitive system of a team of people and the cognitive content that is distributed between individuals. [34, 35] Thus, a key aspect is the process of mutual performance monitoring, where team members monitor each other's activities. Mutual performance monitoring entails the ability to keep track of fellow team members' work, while carrying out one's own work, to ensure that everything is running as expected.[36] This combined awareness of one's own, other team members', and the overall team's situation is elemental to team SA[3].

Managing Technology to Preserve SA

Modern airliners are highly automated. In addition to possessing basic flying skills, it is imperative that pilots are competent technology mangers. They must learn to interface with highly technical systems and equipment, understand how those systems interact with one another, and interpret the data provided by those systems. On the one hand, automated systems support higher levels of SA, reducing task load and freeing up cognitive resource for acquiring and processing information. On the other hand, technology and automation induce a whole new set of vulnerabilities which can drastically reduce SA if not managed appropriately. The modern-day hospital bedside has seen the proliferation of surveillance and monitoring systems that provide us with enormous amounts of patient information. Just as is the case with pilots, nurses must also maintain basic skills while learning to interpret and manage automated systems. To assist nurses in avoiding the technology trap, which can drastically deplete clinical SA, the next section discusses general conceptual philosophies for managing automation.

Reduce levels

One of the interesting things I observed when conducting simulator sessions as an aircrew instructor was the incredible draw that certain pieces of technology created in the cockpit. On the flight deck exists a small computer called a flight management system (FMS). Pilots enter commands into this computer and it tells the aircraft things like where to go, when to turn, and when to start descending. Sometimes, the flight management computer commands the aircraft to do something the pilots are not anticipating or expecting. These can be very tense moments. It usually goes like this: The aircraft fails to turn as expected and you hear someone say, "Hey, what's it doing now?" The "it" of course refers to the computer, which is simply doing what it was told to do. This is when, as a simulator instructor, I would sit back and observe. Pilots who handled this situation well would calmly remove the FMS from the loop, no longer giving it control of the aircraft and then manually assume control of the aircraft. Once this was done, they would correct the problem and then bring the technology back into the equation. This strategy is called reducing levels. Here the pilot reverts to the basics of manual flight and navigation, purposefully ignoring the automation. If this strategy was not employed, the heads of both crew members would go down to the FMS display and that little computer would take the crew deeper and deeper down the road of confusion.

Reducing levels is a great strategy for nurses to remember. Think of all the different values, parameters, and telemetry we can receive from automated physiologic monitoring systems at the bedside. For example, suppose we have a patient who is on a mechanical ventilator on an acute care unit. While in the room with our back to the patient, we hear the ventilator alarm go off. We quickly troubleshoot for leaks, kinks, or obstructions, we check connections and verify settings, but the low-pressure alarm continues to sound. We become suspicious of the machine; we are not sure what the problem is or if the machine is delivering any volume at all. In this situation it is best to stop monkeying around with the ventilator and come down a level. This means we go back to the patient and call on our basic assessment skills to manage the situation. We disconnect the ventilator from the patient, obtain an ambu bag, and ventilate the patient manually. Remember don't let technology take you to a place where your SA becomes dangerously low and you lose the big picture. Always be prepared to momentarily reduce levels.

Verify inputs

Figure 7.4 is a picture of an FMS. Pilots type commands into the keyboard, and the computer follows them. The button that is circled is called the execute button. Once this is pressed, the computer receives and acts on those commands. Before this button is pressed, inputs are verified by two crew members. It is a nonnegotiable standard. One pilot will state what he or she has loaded, and the other crew member follows along and acknowledges agreement. As a rule, the data being entered into this computer is too important to be accomplished unilaterally.

FIGURE
7.4

Flight Management System

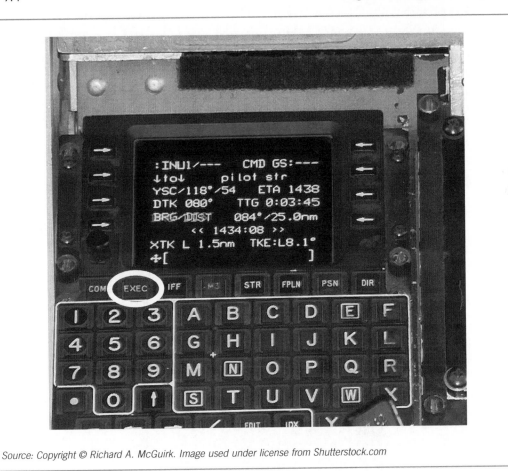

Source: Copyright © Richard A. McGuirk. Image used under license from Shutterstock.com

The FMS looks an awful lot like the infusion pump pictured in Figure 7.5. The pump, like the FMS , has a keyboard; within is a little computer brain that will do what we tell it to do. Circled is the start button that will carry out our commands. In 2006, a patient safety survey of more than 4,800 nurses offered the following statement: I double-check critical medications (such as heparin and vasoactive medications) with another professional before giving them. Barely more than three-quarters acknowledged doing so. A key concern in this survey is that ICU nurses scored well below the mean in this area.[37] Although policies may require double-checks, the culture may be lagging behind. Put simply, with high-risk medications and/or fragile patients, a redundant verification with two staff members must occur before the start button is pressed. While there are many reasons that can be given to say this is unrealistic, such as staffing, workflow issues, and the emergence of smart pumps, utilizing other staff is consistent with the principles of good CRM and provides a last chance to trap errors before they reach the patient.

FIGURE
7.5

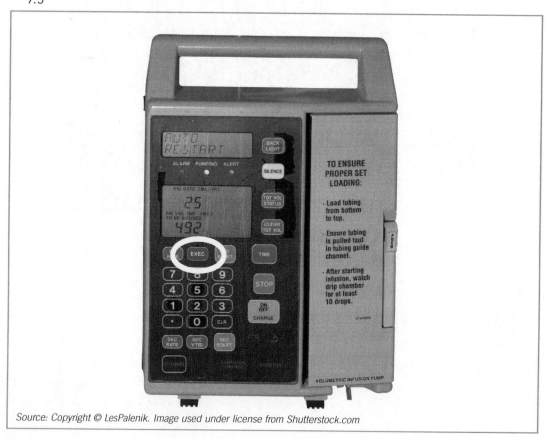

Source: Copyright © LesPalenik. Image used under license from Shutterstock.com

Automated alarms and monitoring systems

There are many monitoring devices in the clinical environment that measure a multitude of physiologic parameters: blood pressure, O_2 saturation, arterial pressure, pulmonary artery pressure, central venous pressure, heart rate, cardiac telemetry, etc. In addition many pieces of biomedical equipment, such as ventilators and dialysis machines, have built-in alarms to warn clinicians of malfunctions. It stands to reason that if the aural alerts and alarms associated with automated monitoring systems are so pervasive in the clinical setting, a discussion of the nurse alarm interface and its potential affect on SA is warranted.

In 2009, the Veterans Administration National Center for Patient Safety published a Patient Safety Advisory highlighting specific examples of patient deaths and close calls associated with physiologic monitoring systems either being turned off or set to inaudible volumes.[38] The advisory provides guidance that suggests never disabling alarms for any reason and ensuring that aural alert volumes are set to at least the manufacturer's default minimum values. Why would patient monitoring equipment ever be set to extremely low volumes or even disabled? We've all heard of alert fatigue.

Working in an environment where there are multiple aural alerts constantly going off makes clinicians weary; eventually, they become desensitized to the alarm and tune it out, turn it down, and in some cases turn it off. In this case the clinician is really saying, "I don't need the alarm, I'll keep my eye on the patient and I'll be able to see if something is wrong."

On the other end of the spectrum of responses exists the opposite of alert fatigue, which is called primary/backup inversion.[40] Here the clinician is saying, "Not only do I depend on the alarm, but I trust the alarm implicitly."

An example of this occurs when a nurse elects to cover up a dialysis access site by placing a blanket on a patient because they are cold. The nurse rationalizes that if the connection with the patient's Permacath™ is disrupted, although the connection is not visible, the danger of exsanguinating is nonexistent because the low-pressure alarm on the dialysis machine will alert her. Unfortunately, we know that patients have exsanguinated from this very situation because the low-pressure alarm either did not go off or did so after the patient lost significant volume. This is the danger with primary/backup inversion; it is a form of complacency where the relationship between human vigilance, which is the primary surveillance system, is switched with automation and technology, which is the backup surveillance system. Making this switch is dangerous because technology and automation can be unpredictable and occasionally fail.

Technology does allow higher levels of SA, and for this reason we should embrace it in patient care. However, we cannot blithely accept that it will always do the right thing and function as advertised. Any situation involving an interface with automation and technology requires continuous monitoring, cross-checking, and evaluation.

On the flight deck, standard operating procedure is that the autopilot will be used for all approaches to airports in low visibility. The pilot shall not hand-fly the aircraft because we know the computer can do it much better than a human being; but it is closely monitored at all times and never trusted implicitly. Attitudes and actions to manage physiologic monitoring systems effectively are:

- Use automation and technology when available

- Automated systems allow for higher levels of clinical SA

- Keep monitoring systems on (unless malfunction is verified)

- Set patient realistic and patient specific alarm parameters to avoid nuisance alerts

- Never disable clinical alarms

- Do not trust monitoring systems implicitly; cross-check with the patient when able

- Always assess the patient; this is the primary detection system

Always follow standard policy and procedure. Bending on standards while thinking that an automated monitoring system will "save me" is setting the stage for poor outcomes.

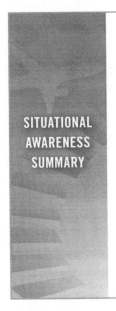

SITUATIONAL AWARENESS SUMMARY

- Know the levels of SA and their application to the clinical decision-making process

- Know the limits of our cognitive resources: attention and working memory

- Identify the threats in the clinical environment that reduce SA

- Adopt countermeasures to maintain higher levels of SA such as:
  - Avoiding premature closure
  - Task load division
  - Maintaining bottom lines
  - Recognizing and resolving red flags

- Adopt attitudes and actions to safely manage automation and technology at the bedside

** NOTE: Other chapters contain strategies that support situational awareness. For an explanation of briefings and shared mental models, see Chapter 5. For an explanation of checklist use and philosophy, see Chapter 9.

References

1.   SA Technologies. n.d. [cited 2010 October 24]; Available from: *http://satechnologies.com/*.

2.   Endsley, M. 1999. Situational awareness in aviation systems. In *Aviation Handbook of Human Factors*, D.J. Garland, J.A. Wise, and V.D. Hopkin, Editors. 1999, Mahwah, NJ: Lawrence Erlbaum Associates.

3.   Salmon, P., N.A. Stanton, and G.H. Walker, and D.P. Jenkins. *Distributed Situation Awareness: Theory, Measurement, and Application to Teamwork* 2009, Burlington, VT: Ashgate.

4.   Dominguz, C. Can SA be defined in *Situation Awareness: Papers and Annotated Bilbliography*, M. Vidulich, et al., Editors. 1994, Wright-Patterson AFB, OH: U.S. Air Force.

5.   Smith, K., and P.A. Hancock. Situation awareness is adaptive, externally directed consciousness *Human Factors, 1995. 37*: p. 137–48.

6.   Endsley, M.R. Towards a theory of situation awareness in dynamic systems. *Human Factors, 1995. 37*(1): p. 32–64.

7.   Khilnani, G.C., and V. Hadda. Management of Severe Sepsis: Role of "Bundles". *The Indian Journal of Chest Diseases & Allied Sciences, 2009. 51*: p. 27–36.

8.   Decker, S., *The Field Guide to Human Error Investigations*. 2002, Burlington, VT: Ashgate.

9.   Saunders, A.F., *Elements of Human Performance: Reaction Processes and Attention in Human Skill*. 1998, Mahwah, NJ: Lawrence Erlbaum Associates.

10. Loukopoulos, L., R. Dismukes, and I. Barshi, *The Multitaskng Myth*. 2009, Burlington, VT: Ashgate.

11. Page, A., ed. *Keeping Patients Safe: Transforming the Work Environment of Nurses*. Institute of Medicine, 2004, Washington, DC: The National Acadamies Press.

12. Meurier, C., C. Vincent, and D. Parmar, Nurses' responses to severity dependent errors: A study of the causal attributions made by nurses following an error *Journal of Advanced Nursing, 1998. 27*: p. 349–354.

13. National Transportation Board, AAR Eastern Alrlines, L-1011, N310EA. 1972: Washington, DC.

14. Reason, J., *The Human Contribution - Unsafe Acts, Accidents, and Heroic Recoveries*. 2008, Burlington, VT: Ashgate.

15. Salvendy, G., ed. *Handbook of Human Factors and Ergonomics*. 3rd ed, ed. G. Salvendy. 2006, Hoboken, NJ: John Wiley and Sons.

16. Gorenflo, D., and J. McConnell, The most frequently cited journal articles and authors in introductory psychology textbooks *Teaching of Psychology, 1991. 18*: p. 8–12.

17. MacLeod, C., and K. Kampe, Word frequency effects on recall, recognition, and word fragment completion tests. *Journal of Experimental Psychology: Learning, Memory, and Cognition, 1996. 22*(1): p. 132–142.

18. Raskin, J., *The Humane Interface.* 2000, Reading, MA: Addison-Wesley.

19. Gobet, F., P.C.R. Lane, P C.H. Cheng, et al., Chunking mechanisms in human learning. *Trends in Cognitive Sciences, 2001. 5*: p. 236–243.

20. Gosbee, J., and L. Gosbee, ed. *Using Human Factors Engineering to Improve Patient Safety.* Oakbrook Terrace, IL: Joint Commission Resources.

21. Klein, G., *Sources of Power: How People Make Decisions.* 1999, Cambridge, MA: MIT Press.

22. Endsley, M.R. T*heoretical Underpinnings of Situational Awareness: A Critical Review in Situational Awareness Analysis and Measurement*, M.R. Endsley and D.J. Garland, Editors. Mahwah, NJ: Lawrence Erlbaum and Associates.

23. Testimony of Captain Sullenberger. 2009. NTSB Public Hearing on the matter of the Landing of US Air Flight 1549 in the Hudson River.

24. Salas, E., et al. Situation awareness in team performance: Implications for measurement and training. *Human Factors: The Journal of the Human Factors and Ergonomics Society, 1995. 37*: p. 123–36.

25. Salas, E., R. Stout, and J.A. Cannon-Bowers. The role of shared mental models in developing shared situational awareness. In *Proceedings of a CAHFA Conference.* 1994, Dayton Beach, FL: Embry-Riddle Aeronautical University Press.

26. Weil, S., P. Foster, J. Freeman, et al. Converging approaches to automated communications-based assessment of team situation awareness, 277–303. In *Macrorecognition in teams*, M. Letsky, N.W. Warner, S.M. Fiore, and C.A.P. Smith, Editors. 2000, Burlington, VT: Ashgate.

27. Gaffney, F.A., S.W. Harden, and R. Seddon. *Crew Resource Management: The Flight Plan for Lasting Change in Patient Safety.* 2005, Marblehead, MA: HcPro, Inc.

28. Vanderbilt University Medical Center. *Crew Resource Management.* Vanderbilt University Medical Center. [cited 2010 10/24]; Available from: *www.mc.vanderbilt.edu/root/vumc.php?site=crew_training&doc=17183/.*

29. Gustafsson, R., et al., *In search of new generation technology programmes.* 2003, Helsinki: Tekes.

30. Ansoff, I., and M. Edward. *Implanting Strategic Management.* 1990, New York: Prentice/Hall.

31. Weick, K., and K. Sutcliffe, *Managning the Unexpected* 2007, San Francisco: Jossey-Bass.

32. Stalhandske, E., The business case for patient safety. *Materials Management in Health Care, 2004. 13*(11): p. 23–37.

33. Weeks, W., J. Waldron, T. Foster, et al. The organizational costs of preventable medical errors. *Journal on Quality Improvement, 2001. 27*(10): p. 533–539.

34. Bartholomew, K. *Ending Nurse-to-Nurse Hostility: Why Nurses Eat Their Young and Each Other.* 2006. Marblehead, MA: HCPro, Inc.

35. Artman, H., and C. Garbis. *Situation awareness as distributed cognition.* In Proceedings of the Ninth European Conference on Cognitive Ergonomics. 1998. Le Chesnay, France.

36. Sonnenwald, D., and L. Pierce. Information behavior in dynamic group work contexts: interwoven situational awareness, dense social and contested collaboration in command and control. *Information Processing and Management, 2000. 36*: p. 461–479.

37. Wilson, K., E. Salas, H.A. Priest, and D. Andrews., Errors in the heat of battle: Taking a closer look at shared cognition breakdowns through teamwork. *Human Factors, 2007. 49*: p. 243–56.

38. The Journal of Clinical Excellence Patient Safety Survey Report. *Nursing, 2006. 5*(5): p. 54–63.

39. VA Headquarters.Alarms On Bedside Physiological Monitors, AD09-09. National Center for Patient Safety 2009 [cited 10/24/2010]; Available from: *www.patientsafety.gov/alerts/AD09-09AudibleAlarmAdvisory.pdf.*

40. Parasuraman, R., et al., Monitoring of Automated Systems, 91–115. In *Automation and Human Performance: Yheory and Applications*, R. Parasuraman and M. Mouloua, Editors. 1996, Mahwah, NJ: p. 91–115.

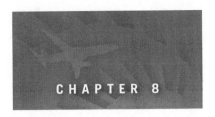

CHAPTER 8

The Sterile Cockpit Concept in Nursing Practice

LEARNING OBJECTIVES

After reading this chapter, the participant will be able to:

- Explain the sterile cockpit principle

- Describe how sterile cockpit principles can be applied to nursing

The previous chapter discussed situational awareness and recognized the complexity of the clinical environment and the competing demands on nurses' attention. This chapter examines strategies for reducing distractions when performing critical tasks.

In 2003, Dr. Theresa Pape, RN, PhD, published a study entitled "Applying airline safety practices to medication administration."[1] For Pape to apply airline cockpit practices in nursing so soon after the release of *To Err is Human*, the Institute of Medicine report that brought patient safety front and center on the national stage, and to do it with such robust research, makes her a visionary in my mind. She is an innovator, willing to think beyond the host of recycled initiatives that have failed to provide nurses with the protections required for safe care during the performance of critical nursing functions.

Her study centered on the idea of using what is called the "sterile cockpit rule" to reduce distractions during medication administration. In the first part of this chapter, I will discuss the sterile cockpit rule and how it plays out in the cockpit and Theresa Pape's 2003 study. In the second part, I will talk about my experiences implementing portions of Pape's work on a large medical–surgical nursing unit. I will discuss how we did this and outline key steps in the process. I'll also highlight the cultural reactions and responses to these implementations—some of which I never expected. Keep in mind that many of the steps described can be applied to any type of unit-based change initiative.

The Sterile Cockpit Rule

Derived from aviation regulations, the sterile cockpit rule (as it is nicknamed) exists to create margins of safety in two ways: First, the rule mandates that pilots not engage in extraneous activity during a critical phase of flight. The critical phase is defined as all operations below an altitude of 10,000 feet, such as taxi, takeoff, and landing. While demand for concentration and multitasking can be present anytime during a flight, operations below 10,000 feet are especially critical because task load, checklist usage, the need for communication both within the cockpit and with air traffic control, and the pace of events all increase sharply. The extraneous activity noted in the rule takes many forms. For example, reading the newspaper; nonessential conversations with flight attendants; idle chitchat within the cockpit such as discussing movies, family, politics, or the latest news; pointing out landmarks to passengers on the public address (PA) system; eating meals—all of these are prohibited during the sterile period. When the cockpit is sterile, pilots must only discuss and engage in the business of operating the aircraft, nothing more. Second, while operating below 10,000 feet, the sterile cockpit rule prohibits employers from requiring flight crews to engage in any company-related duty or activity that is not directly related to the safe operation of the aircraft. Such duties might be promotional PA announcements for the airline, filling out forms or logs, calling ground personnel on the radio to order supplies, or confirming passenger connections.

The rule has teeth. It is a federal regulation and has the full weight of the law behind it. More relevant is the fact that among pilots, the rule is accepted, valued, and practiced. For example, it is not uncommon for one pilot to say to another, "the cockpit is sterile" when miscellaneous nonflying-related comments gain momentum and develop into discussion. The message here is: Let's cut the nonessential chatter and stay focused.

Sadly, there is plenty of supporting evidence in the archives of aviation accidents to demonstrate the consequences resulting from prolonged violation of this rule. One has to look no further than the crash of Continental Connection Flight 3407 outside Buffalo, NY, in February 2009 that killed 50 passengers and crew. While there were other contributing factors identified, the National Transportation Safety Board (NTSB) cited the crew's failure to adhere to sterile cockpit procedures as a causal factor. In the end, the crew failed to monitor the speed of the airplane as they prepared for their approach to the runway. They decelerated below a safe speed and ultimately lost control of the aircraft. In safety-sensitive endeavors, there is little margin for loss of focus.

A key point about the sterile cockpit regulation is the mandate that airlines will not require pilots to perform collateral activities during a critical phase of operation. The onus to avoid distractions is as much on employers of pilots as it is on the pilots themselves. Let's compare this to nursing. As we discussed in Chapter 1, nurses are often pressured or required to perform nonvalue-added, nonessential functions that encroach into critical phases of practice. Case in point, if patient transport is short of personnel, if there is no one in the pharmacy to bring medications to the floor, if housekeeping is running behind and trash needs to be emptied or a spill cleaned up, if a patient needs food and no one is available in dietary to bring it to the floor, then nursing often picks up the slack and sees that these things get taken care of. I want to be clear here: I am not implying that these tasks are not important, because clearly to the patient they are. However, I am saying that often times there is simply no one available to complete such functions and it is culturally acceptable, and often required, that nurses step in and get the job done. This of course comes at a price. When I talk with large groups of nurses, I ask the following question: "What is your primary job as a nurse?" Here is the response I frequently receive: "Everything." This is telling. A group that does everything cannot do anything really well. A nurse's primary job is to assess a patient's condition using specialized education and training, then take that information and use critical thinking to make sound clinical decisions. Nurse leaders must never lose sight of this fact.[2] When nurses are saddled with collateral duties that are not directly related to their primary function, especially during critical times, the risk of patient harm increases and patient safety is compromised. ◆

Remember the example of the pilot helping the flight attendants serve peanuts and soda in Chapter 1? This would

> ◆ Sidebar 8.1
>
> **Task saturation**
>
> Numerous studies have shown that as tasks increase in number, time pressure will cause people to use less of the information available in making their decisions.[3] In times of increased stress, task shedding takes place as low-priority tasks (or steps within tasks) are omitted altogether and speed of task execution is traded against accuracy.[4] As the priority tasks rise to the forefront of prospective memory, cognition, and execution, the "weak signals" of latent errors are missed, misinterpreted, or simplified until a near-miss or a mishap occurs.[5]

be ludicrous and would never happen, but the sterile cockpit regulation does protect pilots form the easy temptation that employers might have to add nonessential duties in the name of efficiency and customer satisfaction. Safety rules. Leaders in healthcare, and especially in nursing, would do well to heed the intent of this part of the sterile cockpit regulation.

The Pape Study

We described the definition of a critical phase of flight for pilots. How about for nurses? What would be considered a "critical phase of practice" for an RN that is worthy of protection from distractions? The answer may depend on the specialty. For example, if you work in an ICU, a critical period may be the first hour of a shift when you are rounding on your patients, performing clinical assessments, tracing infusion lines from the patient to the pump, verifying dosages and infusion rates, and checking ventilator settings. If you work in an oncology area, it may be the period of time where you perform the numerous checks and verifications that accompany the administration of chemotherapy. If you practice on an acute care unit that receives direct admissions, perhaps it is that period of time right after a patient arrives on the unit where a complete evaluation and assessment of the patient must take place. One specific nursing function that cuts across all nursing specialties is medication administration. If you are a practicing nurse of any sort, chances are you will at some time or another be administering medications. Theresa Pape analogized medication administration to the critical tasks performed in the cockpit and set out to study the effect of applying sterile cockpit procedures to medication administration on a medical–surgical nursing unit. This was brilliant and innovative research. Let's look at what Pape accomplished.

In Pape's study, there were three groups. The first was the control group who gave medications normally, or as I say, the old-fashioned way. The second group, called the Focused Protocol group, gave medications using an administration checklist, and had the assistance of fellow staff protecting and shielding the medication nurse from interruptions, running interference and intercepting phone calls where necessary. Behavior modifications were also part of the Focused Protocol. Staff were to avoid interrupting the med nurse, and the med nurse was encouraged to refrain from conversation unless it pertained to the business of passing medications. The third group implemented a MedSafe Protocol. Here nurses gave medications using the checklist, had the benefit of fellow staff shielding and protecting them from distraction, and practiced behavior that avoided extraneous conversation and interruption, but also wore a vest that had the words "MedSafe Nurse: Do Not Disturb" on the front and back. This was a bold step.

It is interesting and humorous to read the discussion in this study. There were some nurses who did not want to take the vest off even after medications had been administered; they wanted to seize the opportunity to continue to get things done without the fits and starts that come with life on the unit. Imagine how much you could accomplish in all phases of life with the use of such a vest. The nurses were observed over eight medication administration events (n = 8) using each protocol and the total number of distractions were tallied for each using a valid and reliable tool called the MADOS (Medication Administration Distraction Observation Sheet).

Here is what Pape discovered (see Figure 8.1). The control group experienced a total of 484 distractions throughout the eight medication passes with an average of 60.5 distractions per pass. The Focused Protocol fared better, reducing distractions to 22.5 per medication pass.

The MedSafe Protocol group experienced a total of 64 observed distractions over the eight medication passes, reducing the mean to eight distractions per pass. Pape demonstrated that nurses can significantly reduce distractions during critical tasks on the nursing unit through the adoption of a sterile cockpit methodology. The corollary to this is of course is that if interruptions and distractions are reduced, medications errors should follow suit.

Figure
8.1

Medication Distractions

Group	Mean	Standard deviation	Total distractions
Control (n = 8)	60.5	12.91	484
Focused protocol (n = 8)	22.5	8.47	180
Medsafe protocol (n = 8)	8.00	4.5	64

Pape explores the idea that we humans are drawn to symbols and that symbols convey meaning. Visible status indicators such as the vest not only demand attention but convey important messages. She discusses the fact that pilots wear wings on their chest and gold stripes on their shoulder. This distinguishes them from other professionals, communicates a level of expertise, and denotes lines of authority. In the same manner, wearing the MedSafe vest achieves the same objective for nurses. It tells others what we do, distinguishes us from other disciplines assigning a commensurate level of expertise, and sends a clear message about how those in our vicinity should respond and interact with us during the medication administration process. In this sense, the vest can be an extremely powerful tool. ◆

◆ Sidebar 8.2
Symbols and influence

Unlike deeper implicit cultural structures such as values and assumptions, explicit observable cultural symbols and behaviors are relatively easy to identify.[6] Unlike memos and vision statements, symbols like the vest and wearing the vest are visible statements that declare the organization is taking overt steps to improve medication and patient safety. In other words, the vest is more than a vest. But the vest must be just one element in an overall strategy used by leaders as they use new stories, new traditions, and new symbols to influence safety culture positively and reduce any perceived ambiguities regarding the priority of medication safety.[7]

Distractions, Interruptions, and Medications

All you have to do is practice nursing on a multibed medical–surgical unit and you understand immediately that interruptions and distractions are commonplace. Based on my experience, I have compiled a list distractions commonly found on the nursing unit. For the nurses out there, see if you agree:

- Loud adjacent conversation

- Multiple people traversing the unit (hospital employees and visitors)

- Questions and requests from visitors

- Requests from physicians

- Fielding phone calls

- Patient call lights

- Ambient noise produced by telephones, fax machines, televisions, and other devices

- Nonnursing functions

- Carts used by various disciplines squealing down the hallway (food and nutrition, housekeeping)

- Maintenance and construction nearby

- Nonessential conversation and interruptions from other nurses

- Cell phones

- Floor buffers

- Resolving missing medications

Soaring to Success

Medication administration requires that nurses interpret prescriber orders, calculate dosages, decipher unfamiliar drug names, reference drug indications, confirm contraindications, cross-check intravenous compatibilities, confirm patient identification, and document appropriately. These requirements are a challenge in any environment but clearly difficult in a setting characterized by the common distractions named above. ◆

◆ Sidebar 8.3

Workplace distractions

In its annual report on medication errors, the United States Pharmacopeia has stated that hospitals cited workplace distractions and interruptions as contributing factors in as high as 47% of all medication errors in hospitals and health systems.[8] A subsequent study asked nurses to rank what they felt were the top 10 reasons why they made medication errors. They ranked the presence of distractions in their environment as the number two cause (poor prescriber handwriting was number one).[9] Clearly, this is a safety-sensitive, complex task, that demands concentration and success. It therefore stands to reason, that to keep patients free from the harm caused by medication-related adverse events, nurses must practice in an environment where distractions, interruptions, and extraneous pressures are substantially mitigated.

A few years ago as a nurse manager of a medical–surgical unit in a large metropolitan hospital, I had the privilege of working with an extremely professional and dedicated group of nurses. As is so often the case, they (we) were struggling with the usual staffing and workload issues that accompany life on the unit. We simply were not going to get more nurses, and when we were well staffed, which was quite often for our unit, nurses would be pulled to other floors, which effectively spread the pain around and just made everyone miserable. The nurse–patient ratios were tough, and we needed to do something different. I wanted to use our resources differently, do something innovative.

With the help of an extraordinary team, we piloted a nursing model that employed solid CRM concepts along with Theresa Pape's sterile cockpit methodology. In the next section I will discuss this experience. This was by no means research; this was messy real-life stuff that was arduous and exhausting, but exciting and rewarding all at the same time. I recently read a quote in a magazine while sitting in the back of an airplane which summed up the entire experience. Christian Haas, group creative director and associate partner for Goody, Silverstein & Partners, when discussing innovation in advertising, said that it:

> *"[O]ften involves approaching advertising differently, taking risks and not doing things that are proven to work. Best practices are by definition the antithesis of innovation, and innovation eventually causes discomfort."*[10]

As you will see, this applies to nursing practice as well as advertising.

Implementing Change: The Real Story

The CRM-based nursing model included three parts: dedicating one nurse solely to the task of medication delivery, implementing an RN to nursing assistant briefing (discussed in Chapter 5), and reducing distractions during medication administration using a variation of Pape's Medsafe protocol. Dedicating a nurse to medication administration and having a patient care nurse who performed assessments and managed care was a departure from the primary care model that we had been using. You might be thinking, "What's the big deal? This is team nursing and has been tried many times before." I would agree. Let's face it; there really is nothing new under the sun.

However, it is completely consistent with CRM, which maximizes human resources to preserve operational safety and efficiency. As we discussed in Chapter 7, dividing the work in this manner ensures that no one person on the team becomes task saturated trying to "do it all." This creates higher levels of team situational awareness (SA), thus increasing the quality of clinical decisions. The Medsafe protocol variation took the form of a vest worn by the medication nurse that read "Do Not Disturb" on the back (See Figure 8.2). The vest was to be worn by the medication nurse during peak medication administration times on the unit. This was the "sterile period."

For example, 9 a.m. was a heavy medication delivery time, so the dedicated med nurse wore the vest from 0800 to 1000. All staff supported the med nurse by shielding and protecting him or her from would-be distracters, and, as in Pape's study, the med nurse was to refrain from engaging in nonessential conversations.

Figure 8.2	Figure 8.3

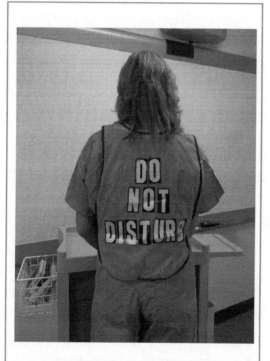

Source: Photo by Gary Sculli. Copyright © 2011.

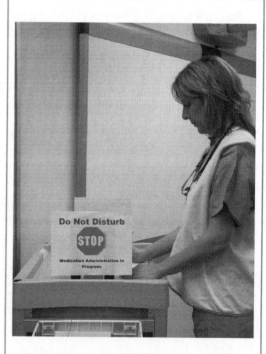

Source: Photo by Gary Sculli. Copyright © 2011.

Getting permission

I was a middle manager, which of course implies pressure from beneath and above. Our unit was stocked with motivated performers hungry to control their own destiny. It was my job to assist and get out of their way, but nothing was going to happen until I had the green light from those who sat above me in the organization. There were two key characters who made all of this possible. The first was my immediate superior, the director of medical–surgical nursing, and the second was the chief nursing officer (CNO). My boss was an innovative spirit who had infectious energy and a formidable mind. ◆

> ◆ Sidebar 8.4
>
> ## Innovation
>
> From a purely business perspective, innovation in organizations is defined as using ideas to create capital. However, for our purposes a better definition is the use of ideas to add *value*. And, despite the current popular literature regarding innovative organizations, it must be remembered that organizations don't innovate … people do. People who innovate may be described as supporting the goals of an organization but having an interest in finding an alternative means to reaching those goals through non-pathological deviation from the norm.[11] Often, the innovator wants a new definition of the problem as well as new solutions. A manager should articulate the vision and goals and then give the employee the space needed to be creative and not overmanage and get in the way of the creative process.
>
> The activities that support innovation involve risk, uncertainly, and even failure. The organization should be prepared to accept failures, because not all innovative ideas are going to be successful. But, like all failures, innovative failures should be used to further other ideas that have a potential for success. Sometimes, it is as valuable to find out what doesn't work as what does.

She walked very fast and had an incredible knack for creatively solving complex problems. When I brought the idea to her, she responded with something like, "Let's do it, man," and she never looked back. Although there were requirements to keep things budget neutral and to have a well-thought-out measurement plan, her support never wavered. Never. The CNO was a principled leader whom I respected greatly. What stands out for me here is that, in conversations with her, I came to understand that she was not a big fan of the movement to bring aviation concepts into nursing practice, yet she supported our efforts through word and action. Here is a nurse leader who was willing to put her own views aside and support a large group of nurses in the name of innovation and autonomy. The CNO provided human resources to help us with literature searches, gave us face time with hospital leaders and other groups to brief them on the project, and publicly praised our efforts to take on ambitious endeavors while still running a very busy medical–surgical nursing unit. Job satisfaction for nurses is directly related to autonomy in practice.[12] Here were two nurse leaders who understood that fact. They provided guidance, support, and resources and then stood aside and let the frontline staff carry the ball. Now that's leadership!

Preparation

I first brought the idea to the staff at a monthly staff meeting. I discussed all facets of the model, but of course much of the discussion gravitated to the sterile cockpit component. When I pitched the MedSafe vest, I think they thought I was truly insane. This type of implementation was not as common as it might be today. There was uncomfortable silence and laughter. I then gave them copies of Pape's study, and we began to have a dialogue. They all agreed that the practice environment on the unit was replete with distractions and interruptions, which made it extremely difficult to administer medications safely and efficiently. What I wanted them to understand was that things could be different; they could change their environment and they were empowered to do so. I wanted them know that their work was worthy of being elevated and protected, and that it was not acceptable for a nurse to be a moving target for anyone to approach while standing in front of a medication cart or in a medication room. Medication administration is, after all, a critical task, completely analogous to a pilot taking off in a fully loaded airplane. It was easy to get agreement on this point. The challenge was moving to the next level: a clear vision that things could be different.

The first step was to identify a core group of nursing staff that were high performers and informal leaders who were motivated to pilot something new. This group represented our "change team" and was easy to find on our unit. We were sure to include all representative players on the team, RNs, licensed practical nurses (LPN), nursing assistants, and unit secretaries. There were several pieces of information we really needed to have before we moved forward and implemented the model. First, we wanted to understand fully the clinical service and function of our unit. What was our most common diagnosis, how many medications did we administer in a day or month, how many admissions and discharges did we average in a day, how many peripherally inserted central catheter (PICC) lines did we manage, and what type of surgical procedures were recovered on the unit? Because we had LPNs on staff and they would primarily be assigned as medication nurses, we wanted to determine whether this would be workable given the restrictions on their practice regarding IV push

◆ Sidebar 8.5
Research or QI?

Was this study research that, because human subject were involved, required review by the local IRB and patient consent or was it simply quality improvement (QI)? Research typically means activities independent of routine medical care undertaken to gain generalizable knowledge and that often include third-party funding and randomization of study subjects that may raise ethics questions. The definition in the Department of Health and Human Services regulations state that "research means a systematic investigation, including research development, testing and evaluation, designed to deliver or contribute to generalizable knowledge."[13]

The Hastings Center notes that QI, on the other hand, "is marked most distinctly by the prompt feedback of the effects of deliberate changes to the same care delivery setting that is making the changes."[14] The vest study was, therefore, simply good clinical care combined with systematic learning to improve medication administration safety and staff performance, and not the type of research that requires IRB review and approval.

medications, use of central lines, and the administration of blood products. We needed to investigate and quantify these activities. One nurse with a particular talent for mining data dutifully and methodically completed this research and prepared a summary report for the rest of the change team. The results looked promising; nothing jumped out at us and said, "This won't work," so we concluded that our unit would be a good match for the model. ◆

Initially, the plan was to implement the model on one side of the unit, which included 20 beds. Our unit had heavy medication volumes; therefore, we had to answer the following question: Was it possible for the medication nurse to deliver all medications to 20 patients within the specified time frame (one hour before to one hour after scheduled delivery time) in a safe manner that did not cause him or her to feel rushed, anxious, or task saturated.

After great debate and discussion, the way we chose to settle this question was to try it! If it didn't work, then we would have to reevaluate.

A key part of the preparation was the focus group meetings. Here we pulled the frontline change team together along with our director and resources provided by the CNO. We outlined the model, discussed pros and cons, and presented variations on how it might play out on the unit. We discussed where and when RN-led briefings would take place, and we debated what the "Do Not Disturb" vest should look like and when it should be worn. We examined past experiences with team nursing that those on the team had experienced, and thoroughly reviewed current literature that related to our implementation. One of the things the group did was something called a "tabletop" exercise. When this was first suggested, I thought to myself, this is silly and would be better suited as a kindergarten exercise. I was wrong. The tabletop exercise was extraordinarily valuable and enabled us to preempt many operational snafus. I sincerely believe the time that we invested in this exercise on the front end made implementation much easier, and I highly recommend this activity for any nursing team attempting to implement change. Here is how it worked for us:

The entire team sat around the table and we started to imagine what the model would look like from beginning to end, down to the smallest detail. Someone would start the discussion, and other people would chime in with their thoughts and observations. In a sense it was a mental simulation. For example we would start by saying,

"At 0645, the nurses will clock in and go to the nurse's station for report."

Then someone else would ask: "What about the Med Nurse? Should she go to report or instead start reviewing medication administration records and setting up carts for the Med Pass?"

This prompted discussion and debate which led to resolution: The Med Nurse would not attend change-of-shift report.

From here the natural question was how will the Med Nurse be made aware of significant information affecting medication delivery such as NPO status and vital signs?

The team then exchanged more ideas and arrived at a conclusion: The RN, in addition to briefing the nursing assistant, would also brief the Med Nurse, covering patient-specific medication-related information.

More questions:

"Would the requirement for the RN to complete two briefings after change-of-shift report create a problem?"
"Where on the unit should the briefing take place so it would not be interrupted?"
"Who would answer call lights during the briefings?"

Other questions emerged:

"Who will administer as-needed (PRN) medications?"
"If a medication order is changed, how will that information be communicated between the RN, Med Nurse, and Unit Secretary?"
"Does the Med Nurse perform glucose measurements as well as administer insulin, or does he or she just administer insulin?"
"What will the Med Nurse do after all patients have received their medications?"
"When does the Med Nurse go to lunch and who will relieve him or her?"

We answered all of these questions and created a strategy to deal with each. The tabletop exercise allowed us to identify and resolve operational issues that we otherwise would not have considered individually prior to implementation. It caused us to discuss strategy and consider contingencies if things started falling apart. It also allowed us to construct a working timeline of the model and establish processes and responsibilities at a granular level.

While nothing we decided was written in stone, and midcourse corrections were necessary, ultimately this exercise removed many obstacles that would have confounded and confused us all in the heat of battle.

"Just do it"

Prior to the focus group meetings with frontline staff, of which there were approximately four, there were at least that many exploratory meetings with just leadership present. All of this was behind us now. We had already determined that no scope of practice guidelines would be violated, that we were not placing patients at risk, and we had a willing and ready frontline change team in place. We had done our due diligence to prepare for implementation of the model. I generally do not have an affinity for meetings and prefer action over prolonged discussion. Others on the team felt the same way. At one point, we just looked at each other and said, "Let's just do it." The night before the first implementation, we pulled the change team together, conducted a short briefing, and made the necessary assignment changes to implement the CRM-based care delivery model on half of the unit.

Over time the model underwent tweaks and adjustments, which produced subtle variations. Before we highlight some of the findings and lessons learned, I would like to discuss the cultural reaction and challenges experienced during the implementation. With all of our preparation, nothing could have prepared us for this. Most of this will center on the use of sterile cockpit procedures during medication administration. Who would have thought a simple little vest with stick-on letters would cause such a stir?

Cultural Reaction

Opposite effect

Even though I briefed hospital service line leadership on what we would be doing on our unit, it was obvious that the message did not get through or was not retained by employees throughout the hospital. From physicians to dietitians to respiratory therapists to chaplains, all had a similar reaction to the "Do Not Disturb" Vest. They would see the nurse wearing the orange vest engrossed in the duties of medication administration, wrinkle their brow, and approach while saying something like, "Do not disturb, what's that all about?" and in the course of doing so would disturb the nurse. People were so curious and thunderstruck that they did not process and therefore obey the clear directions on the vest; they had to ask questions.

Quite honestly, in the beginning, this was a real problem and affected the staff's perception of the vests' effectiveness. Even if the nurse tried to ignore their queries, if no one was immediately there to intercept the disruption, it made for some awkward moments. I did not anticipate this. What I found to be an absolute necessity was that my presence was constantly required on the unit early on in the implementation to assist with protecting the staff and educating those who were curious. I made at least a hundred copies of the Theresa Pape article and as I explained to onlookers what we were doing, I would give them a copy to read. No doubt that the vest is a bold statement, and I wanted it that way. I wanted people to know what these nurses were doing and why. However, with that came a spike of queries and unsolicited opinions, which increased distractions and interruptions. Over time this got much better, but initially it was difficult to manage and tested our resolve. I am glad we persevered.

Other disciplines: Pushback

Everyone was curious, but there were some who had an opinion about the sterile cockpit initiative and were not afraid to say it. In other words, there were detractors among us. Not agreeing or seeing the value in this project is fine with me, because everyone is entitled to their opinion; however, when critics become hecklers, it needs to be dealt with immediately. Change implementation can easily be derailed in the early stages by this sort of behavior. There were three encounters that I remember quite clearly. One involved an individual who was not a nurse and worked in another discipline. The staff was concerned that his vocal opposition to the vest out on the unit was becoming a problem. I asked him to come to my office so we could discuss the matter. He told me that in his opinion it was not morally acceptable for a nurse to tell a patient that he or she was not available, and it sent the wrong message to those we cared for. My immediate response to him was, "Do medication errors send the right message to patients?" "Why is it not acceptable for a nurse to deflect nonemergent requests in order to stay focused on a critical safety-sensitive task"? We debated and discussed the issue, but in the end agreed to disagree. I respected this individual's point of view; people are passionate about their beliefs, especially when patients are involved, but I wanted him to cease the vocal opposition to the project while out on the unit, which he agreed to do. For me this reaction was interesting and indicative of a pervasive phenomenon. When nurses boldly exert control over their practice environment, people seem to get nervous. Interesting.

The second encounter involved a nonclinical nurse that was often present on our unit. She was not part of our staff, but did interact frequently with our nurses. Again I was informed that this person was stridently voicing negative opinions about the model while working at the nurses' station. Her issues were somewhat different. In her mind she felt that the vest was demeaning, that it was unprofessional and made the nurse look like a construction worker. I truly did not know what to say in response. In one sense she was correct. In fact the orange vests in the first phase of the pilot most likely were procured from construction surplus. To make matters worse, the letters were stick-on, like the ones you put on a mailbox. Was this really important? The purpose of the implementation is to focus on distractions, not fashion. While the vest was not perfect, and we clearly had all intentions of changing it to a more permanent design, it was aesthetically acceptable and certainly not meant to demean anyone. The nurses on our unit were not shy; if it was not at least acceptable, they would have rejected it outright. This reaction speaks to the constant requirement to keep detractors focused on the fundamentals, which are enhanced levels of safety and reduced risk of harm to patients.

The third encounter involved a "sitter" who was an unlicensed agency nurse employed not by the hospital, but by one particular patient's family to sit with the patient at all times. This sitter, an elderly woman, parked herself in the doorway to the patient's room so she could watch the patient as well as the activity in the hall. One day, as our Medication Nurse was leaving the room, the sitter stood up and quite loudly asked herself, "Do not disturb"? "Since when is it that we aren't allowed to disturb a nurse?" Again, education was required and offered.

I was encouraged by the reactions we received from the physicians who regularly admitted patients to the unit. In my conversations with them, they exhibited sincere interest in all facets of the model (teamwork to enhance situational awareness, briefings, and sterile cockpit protocols) and supported what we were trying to accomplish. While I was not privy to all conversations they had with the staff during normal operations, I received no reports, nor did I personally experience pushback or protest from the physician group. It was my impression that they were in favor of any initiative that aimed to increase the level of safety for their patients.

Sterile Cockpit Vest, Verbiage, and Signs

I soon learned that when it comes to a sterile cockpit implementation, not any old vest will do. Discussion and debate about what the optimal vest should look like continued well into the implementation. The first vest was bright orange and had the words "Do Not Disturb" on the back. Many of the staff who wore the vest started to feel as though the words were too direct. The consensus was that the vest was harsh and might be offending people with its verbiage. To quote a former president, we needed something "kinder and gentler." We put a second vest into service and this time it read "Please Do Not Disturb." Everyone felt better.

Later we used a yellow vest that had no words at all. The Med Nurse wore the vest all of the time and it served the sole purpose of signifying his or her function on the team. This was significant because we wanted to emphasize the task load division element of the model. On the Med Cart we placed signs reading "Do Not Disturb - Medication Administration in Progress" (See Figures 8.2 and 8.3). The signs were removable and placed in position only when medications were being delivered. This is consistent with a second study by Theresa Pape in 2005 that used "Do Not Disturb" signs in lieu of a vest. We wanted to combine Pape's two methodologies. As the nurse moved from room to room wearing the yellow vest, with signs in place on each side of the Med Cart, it was though she had created a literal cockpit for herself. This worked quite well.

Soaring to Success

The vest we ultimately settled on was chosen by the staff and procured from a reputable vendor rather than construction surplus. To get to this point, we had to consider many variables and learn by trial and error.

Nurses

Andrew McVicar, BSc, PhD, in his discussion of workplace stress in nursing, states the following:

> Moves during the 1980s and 1990s to promote a more holistic approach to care have altered the dynamic between nurses and patients, from one in which nurses might distance themselves from the emotional needs of patients to one in which development of a nurse–patient relationship is considered essential. Such 'emotional labor' places considerable demands on those delivering health care and may reduce objectivity in caring.[15]

In addition to knowing a vast amount of technical knowledge, a significant facet of professional nursing involves the "art" of caring. This is what sets nursing apart from other disciplines. Nurses form bonds with their patients; they say just the right thing at the right time to calm someone who is frightened about a procedure or a devastating diagnosis. Nurses hold a hand or touch a shoulder to comfort the dying, or soothe a family member who has lost a loved one. With this, however, comes the emotional labor that McVicar discusses. It is in the professional culture to "be there" for our patients, no matter what. To say "I'm not available" is in many cases anathema to nurses. The problem is that it's not possible to be available to everyone all of the time for everything and still have operational success at tasks requiring thought work and careful concentration. Other industries have figured this out; why not ours?

Nurses were now asked to be completely objective and somewhat removed with regard to an aspect of patient care, and it was clearly putting pressure on long-held cultural paradigms.

Each time we implemented the model, the staff would assemble after the shift for a debriefing. It was in the debriefing where we identified what was working, what was not working so well, and what adjustments were necessary. A frequent topic in the debriefing concerned the degree to which the Med Nurse should be removed from responding to patient needs and requests. We created some guidelines, but left the rest up to individual judgment.

For example, if the Med Nurse sees that a patient is hanging over the side rail about to fall out of bed or an emergency situation exists, than clearly this would not be the time to turn away and say, "Sorry, I'd love to help but I can't be disturbed." There is not a nurse on the planet who would do such a thing, so this was an easy guideline to set. The difficulty came when discussing more subtle situations like nonemergent questions and requests from patients or family members. A nurse standing in front of Med Cart is often the most visible when peering down the corridor of a nursing unit and is a natural target when someone is searching for a nurse, or anyone for that matter. The fact that other team members were actively shielding and protecting the Med Nurse helped, but it wasn't always effective.

One of the tools we developed were short scripts that the Med Nurse could use in response to requests that would politely deflect the distraction. The bottom line here is that whatever is decided, the spirit and intent of the sterile cockpit implementation need to be preserved. If the line gets too blurry, then the critical task of medication administration is no longer adequately protected. Some nurses could see the line very clearly, while others had trouble. This is something we revisited often throughout the pilot.

Earlier I mentioned that when the concept of the vest was pitched to the staff, there was laughter and uncomfortable silence. After a while, the nurses warmed up to the idea of the vest and the sterile cockpit concept. As the pilot progressed, I truly enjoyed watching many nurses freely don the "Do Not Disturb" vest and proceed with their work while others intercepted distractions and interruptions. It truly was a team effort and a thing of beauty when all cylinders were firing smoothly. Some nurses would say, "I was vest on" or "I was vest off" when describing what they were doing at a particular time. It was becoming a part of their language and routine. I would be lying if I said there weren't resisters, but they were few.

Patients

When we piloted the care delivery model, patients were briefed at the beginning of the shift that they would have two nurses, one who would provide and manage their care, and another who would be administering their medications. They were also briefed on the reason for the vest. This was accomplished on beginning-of-shift rounds by both the primary care nurse and the Med Nurse. In our postimplementation debriefings, nurses would frequently report that patients were pleased with the fact that they got to have "two nurses today." They relayed many positive comments made by patients about having more face time with nurses as well as the efforts to reduce distractions in the interest of safety. I was not aware of any patient complaints about what we were doing.

Lessons Learned

Here, I present a summary of lessons learned as we moved through the process of implementing this CRM-based care delivery model. While we gained much knowledge from this experience, I have narrowed it down to a handful of key points:

Change is messy

When you read a paper or research study, it all sounds so tidy and controlled, but I hardly think this reflects reality. Even with months of preparation and planning, when an innovative project is turned loose on the unpredictable and capricious realm of human beings, anything is possible. As the steward of a project, you have a blueprint in your mind as to how things will proceed; however, you have to be flexible and understand that things rarely follow such a blueprint. There needs to be a few nonnegotiable concepts and principles that keep an implementation on track, but how the final product will ultimately look is rarely known early on. As the leader of change you have to be open-minded, allowing for the influence of the many competing goals and backgrounds that human beings carry with them. You must also be willing to accept that success may look completely different from what you first imagined.

Be bold

If you want to make a statement, you cannot be timid. For example, recall the initial vest that we used: bright orange with stick-on letters. This was an audacious move on our part and quite frankly was by design. We wanted to challenge long-held paradigms regarding the behavioral expectations of professional nurses; to do so it was necessary to get people's attention. I am not suggesting the use of hokey schemes for shock value; this hurts credibility. I am suggesting that if you have done good research and due diligence, and you believe in the concept, take it to the limit and do not let detractors take the wind out of your sails. For example, when I talk with nursing units today about how best to implement a version of Pape's MedSafe protocol, my advice is use both the vest and signs, not one or the other.

Initial presence is required

During implementation of the pilot, my presence as the leader of the unit was constantly required for two main reasons. The first was to deal with the education of curious onlookers and detractors who were creating "noise." The second was to talk with the staff to reinforce agreed upon processes and offer miscellaneous assistance. Over time, however, the requirement for my presence diminished as processes became more established. Constant presence became regularly scheduled rounding, which ultimately went to occasional rounding on the unit. At the end of the pilot, my presence was not required.

High performers and change team

Not to be cliché, but human beings hate change. When implementing change, especially change that directly challenges current practice, you want to set yourself up for success. For this reason, we chose motivated clinicians with a history of strong performance: "high performers." We also tried to include those that would be considered informal leaders on the unit, those that had the ability to sway others by what they did and said. There is nothing wrong with manipulating the process in this manner. As expected, our initial implementations went extraordinarily well. As we spread the implementation and got deeper into the staff roster, things quite frankly at times looked ugly. I will never forget the day I decided to round on the unit during an afternoon medication pass. As I looked down the hall I saw the Med Nurse wearing the vest, her head cocked to the side leaning against the wall having what was clearly a flirtatious conversation with a young gentleman. This was not exactly required communication. You have to be prepared for added oversight and reinforcement as you get further away from the highest performers. You must also accept that what you encounter there most closely resembles reality.

Debriefing

Each day after we implemented the model, we had a debriefing with the participating staff. This lasted anywhere from 10–30 minutes, although we tried to keep it short. The purpose was to review what was working and what needed to be improved or changed. We did this without exception, and it should always be included in any unit-based pilot or trial. We were also able to use the debriefing as an opportunity to measure and record staff perceptions about the model. This was accomplished by administering a Likert scale questionnaire to participants, which was later replaced with guided oral questioning to identify specific themes in the staff responses.

Nurses won't let go

I remember my conversation with one nurse in particular, a superb and dedicated clinician in every respect and holder of an advanced degree. She was simply not comfortable letting the Med Nurse administer medications and was having intense difficulty letting go of this task. Even though she had a complete list of medications that were being administered for her reference, she was not comfortable unless she physically prepared, then handed the medications to the patient. We debated and discussed this, but I could see this was a major problem for her. Recall in Chapter 5 where I discussed the reaction to the RN to Nursing Assistant Briefing Checklist; some nurses could not get used to using a checklist to guide communication routinely and felt silly doing so. These observations are not criticisms, simply realities. Although there were aspects of the model these nurses valued and accepted, there were others with which they would comply, but never fully accept. Fair enough.

Communication

As discussed in Chapter 7, silos themselves aren't bad, but silos with poor communication are. Any time you implement a care delivery model that divides up tasks the need for communication increases. One of the things we developed early (the tabletop helped with this) was a communication process. It was essentially a hub-and-spoke communication model. Since the RN was directing and managing patient care, all communication had to be brought back to him or her (the hub), then go out to the rest of the team (the spokes).

Leadership

For an implementation like this to be successful, higher level leadership must be aware and support it. Support can come in many forms. In some organizations the CNO may openly champion the innovative change and attend meetings with staff. In others, leadership may simply require occasional updates of progress, agreeing not to micromanage the situation. On our unit, the presence of the Medical Surgical Director at all front line meetings along with the resources and open support provided by the CNO, spoke volumes to the staff. Ultimately though, it's up to the front line manager to effectively make the case for change and garner leadership support.

FIGURE
8.4

Aggregate Results

Here are the results from the debriefing questionnaire (n = 68):

This model improved teamwork.

32% agree strongly
53% agree
12% neutral
3% disagree
n/a disagree strongly

This model allowed for the RN to spend more time on patient assessments.

35% agree strongly
47% agree
16% neutral
1% disagree
n/a disagree strongly

The "Do Not Disturb" vest along with teamwork served to reduce distraction during peak medication administration times.

26% agree strongly
48% agree
22% neutral
1% disagree
1% disagree strongly

The division of tasks in the model did not reduce my ability to remain informed about my patient.

16% agree strongly
46% agree

31% neutral
6% disagree
1% disagree strongly

This model improved communication between the nursing assistant and nurse.

34% agree strongly
51% agree
13% neutral
1% disagree
n/a disagree strongly

Other healthcare workers were accepting of this model.

16% agree strongly
56% agree
25% neutral
3% disagree
n/a disagree strongly

This model allowed for the safe delivery of medications to patients.

31% agree strongly
49% agree
19% neutral
1% disagree
n/a disagree strongly

Note: Percentages are cumulative. Rounding may cause the sum of total percentages to be < 100%.

COMMON THEMES

The following common themes emerged from postimplementation debriefings.

Positive:

- More time available to spend with patients, talk with physicians

- Unhurried and more thorough patient assessments

- Fewer call lights, less noise

- Less stress, calmer unit environment

- Nurse-to-nursing assistant briefing enhanced communication

- Meds delivered more efficiently

Negative:

- Giving medications and not having the complete patient picture

- Managing care and not having complete patient picture

- Model is very dependent on good communication

- Communication breakdowns can cause things to be missed

Other results during model implementation:

- Falls – no increase (falls consistent with previous periods)

- Medication variances – none reported (consistent with previous periods)

- Incidental – 2.7% increase in patient discharges before noon

- Patient satisfaction – While this was not research and there was no control, it piques interest to note that, during model implementation, there was a marked increase in Mean Patient Satisfaction scores

References

1. Pape, T.M., Applying airline safety practices to medication administration. *Medsurg Nursing, 2003. 12*(2): p. 77–93.

2. Institute of Medicine, *Keeping Patients Safe: Transforming the Work Environment of Nurses*, ed. A. Page, Washington, DC: The National Academies Press.

3. Payne, J.W., J.R. Bethman, and E.J. Johnson, Adaptive strategy reflections in decision making. *Journal of Experimental Psychology, Learning, Memory, and Cognition, 1988. 14*: p. 534–52.

4. Mackenzie, C., S. Jeffcott, and Y. Xiao. Measuring the Impact of Time Pressure on Team Task Performance, in *Safer Surgery: Analysing Behavior in the Operating Theater,* R. Flin and L. Mitchell, Editors. 2009, Burlington, VT: Ashgate.

5. Weick, K., and K. Sutcliffe, *Managing the Unexpected* 2007, San Francisco: Jossey-Bass.

6. Schein, E.H., *Organizational Culture and Leadership.* 3rd ed. 2004, San Francisco: Jossey-Bass. 370.

7. National Defense University. *Strategic Leadership and Decision Making.* n.d. [cited 8/11/2010]; Available from: *www.au.af.mil/au/awc/awcgate/ndu/strat-ldr-dm/cont.html.*

8. U.S. Pharmacopeia. Summary of information submitted to Medmarx in the year 2002: Quest for Quality. 2003. [cited 8/10/2010]; Available from: *www.usp.org/pdf/EN/medmarx/2002MEDMARXSummary.pdf.*

9. Mayo, A.M., and D. Duncan. Nurse Perceptions of Medication Errors: What We Need to Know for Patient Safety. *Journal of Nursing Care Quality:, 2004. 19*(3): p. 209–217.

10. Elbert, S. The Mad Mad World of Advertising. *Delta Sky Magazine, July 2010:* p. 60–67.

11. Merton, R.K. *Social Theory and Social Structure.* 1968, New York: Free Press.

12. Zangaro, G.A., and K.L. Soeken. A meta-analysis of studies of nurses' job satisfaction. *Research in Nursing and Health, 2007. 30*(4): p. 445–58.

13. U.S. Department of Health & Human Services. Code of Federal Regulations: Protection of Human Subjects. Section 46.102(d). [cited 8/12/2010]; Available from: *www.hhs.gov/ohrp/humansubjects/ guidance/45cfr46.htm#46.102.*

14. Baily, M., M. Bottrell, J. Lynn, and B. Jennings, *The Ethics of Using QI Methods to Improve Health Care Quality and Safety.* 2006, The Hastings Center.

15. McVicar, A. and Journal of Advanced Nursing, 2003. 44(6): p. 633–642

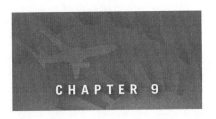

CHAPTER 9

Developing Checklists on the Nursing Unit

LEARNING OBJECTIVES

After reading this chapter, the participant will be able to:

- Explain how checklists improve patient safety

- Describe strategies for using checklists in the nursing environment

In Chapter 1, we made the point that checklists are a staple in the airline industry, perhaps the backbone of the cockpit safety culture. We also made the point that pilots discipline themselves to use checklists as part of standard procedures and they do so without question. Yes, there are times, especially in emergency or abnormal scenarios, where a pilot must apply judgment by deciding what checklist to use or whether a step within the checklist is truly appropriate, but to disregard a checklist entirely is extremely rare and completely deviant.[1]

Checklists are not new to nursing. In some variation or another, we have all used them in practice. Earlier I challenged you to think back over your professional career and remember a time where you used a checklist in patient care. Was it easy to use? Did it make sense? Did it make your job easier or create more work for you? These are important questions. Checklists function to support human memory; they place knowledge in the world so you don't have to keep it in your head.[2] Checklists also support situational awareness (SA) by directing our assessments so we pay attention to the right things at the right time. ◆

If, however, checklists are not used properly, and more importantly, if they are not *developed* properly:

- They will **not** be easy to use

- They will **not** make sense

- They will **not** make your job easier

- They **will** create more work for you

◆ Sidebar 9.1

Interruptions and checklists

Recognizing the risks associated with task interruption and the weaknesses of prospective memory (i.e., remembering to resume an interrupted task) can lead to better task management and an increased awareness of the prototypical situations that are prone to unwelcome and unwanted task interruption (e.g., medication administration). Such awareness can help identify good stopping points in critical tasks, to develop strategies to deal with the inevitable interruption, and also to clarify when and how to interrupt others engaged in critical tasks when an interruption is absolutely necessary. A checklist can be used after a task is interrupted to either return to the next step in the task or as a visual reminder to return to the beginning of the task.[3]

I think back to my days on the med–surg unit as a staff nurse, busily caring for a group of patients and getting the call to premedicate and send a patient to surgery. I would reference the preoperative checklist located at the front of the chart. If it was a good day and I was ahead of the game, most of the items on the checklist had been completed well before the moment the operating room called for the patient. However, I admit there were instances where this was not the case and I would find that only a few items had been addressed, or worse yet, none of the items had been addressed. It was times like this I really needed the checklist to be simple, concise, and clear. This wasn't the case. The checklist was exceedingly long and had excessive verbiage. Some items required me to fill in a blank; other parts required me to answer yes or no questions, then presented me with actions based on my answer. Some items seemed superfluous and nonapplicable. For me, using this checklist was a cognitive nightmare and getting through it was like swimming in glue, always getting bogged down on some granular detail. As is often the case when human beings achieve miserable results attempting to use a tool that is not well constructed, I blamed myself.

Obviously, I had some kind of cognitive processing deficiency that was only now surfacing in adulthood. As I would learn years later from my experience using checklists in the cockpit, the problem was not me; it was the checklist.

Checklist Philosophy

In nursing we often see checklists in the form of order sets, flow sheets, protocols, cognitive aids, care plans, and algorithms. Although designed with good intent, these tools often have limited usability and differ significantly from airline style checklists.[4] In the cockpit, checklists are developed to fit specific operations. How checklists are presented and what they look like are predicated on how the flight crew will actually use them in each situation. When developing and using checklists in nursing practice, the same considerations should apply. Checklists can be divided into two types: **read and verify** and **read and do**. Let's look at each.

Read and verify checklists

Read and verify checklists are used for normal procedures. Normal procedure means anything that is done consistently and repeatedly on a routine basis, most often from memory. For example a pilot learns where to position certain switches and controls for takeoff, something he will do multiple times in a day. The pilot completes the actions from memory, and then references the checklist to verify that nothing is missed. For nurses, normal procedures analogous to takeoff for the pilot could be setting up an infusion pump, starting an IV, passing medications, or doing preoperative teaching. The key point about the read and verify checklist is that a series of steps are first completed from memory, then the checklist is read as a final step to back up and support human memory.

One thing to keep in mind with read and verify checklists is that if they are to be used in the manner described, particular attention must paid to how information is presented to the user. Figure 9.1 is a generic example of a read and verify checklist used in aviation prior to takeoff. Disregard the aviation content and focus in on the way the checklist appears. On the left side of the checklist, there are nouns that tell the reader what item requires an action. On the right, there are either verbs in the past tense, indicating that something has already been accomplished, or there are a few words describing the condition or placement of a switch. Notice that the checklist is not loaded with narrative or expanded verbiage. It is presented in a manner that is simple, uncluttered, and easy to read. The checklists items are clear and concise, allowing ease of use.

FIGURE
9.1

Read and Verify Checklist

Before Takeoff

Window Heat...ON HIGH
Anti-Ice.. ON
Flight Instruments & Radios.. SET
Yaw Damper...ON & CHECKED
Flight Controls..CHECKED
Stabilizer Trim .... SET
Flaps / Slats .... 15 & GREEN
Electrical..NO LIGHTS
Fuel Pumps... SET FOR TAKEOFF
Fuel Heat ....OFF
Hydraulics... PRESS & QTY NORMAL
Elevator & Rudder Lights ....OFF
Air Cond & Press.. SET FOR TAKEOFF
EPR & Airspeed Bugs.. SET
Transponder ....ALTITUDE
Takeoff Briefing ....COMPLETE

There are many normal processes and procedures in nursing that can benefit from the use of a well-constructed read and verify checklist. As an example, let's take the task of starting an IV and hanging a 1-L bag of normal saline to run at a specified rate. This is a normal procedure, something nurses do all of the time, perhaps several times in a day or week. They are very familiar with the task and while attention is required, the steps and actions in the process can be completed without intense focus and concentration. I can picture an experienced nurse preparing supplies, prepping the skin, inserting the IV catheter, dressing the site, and hanging the infusion while at the same time talking with the patient or the patient's family about a medication or upcoming surgery. The nurse has done this so many times she can do it without thinking. ◆

This is the perfect situation for a read and verify checklist. If you are a nurse you might ask, "Why would I need a checklist in this situation? I do this all of the time and I don't see the benefit." I would urge you to stop for a moment and answer the following questions: Have nurses ever forgotten to remove tourniquets after venipuncture, only to be discovered hours later? Have nurses ever started an IV in an arm that is contraindicated because of an arterial-venous graft or potential lymphedema

---

◆ Sidebar 9.2

What is attention, exactly?

"Everyone knows what attention is," began a passage by William James in *Principles of Psychology* that is often referred to by cognitive psychologists as they grope to describe attention. James continues, attention is "the taking possession of the mind, in clear and vivid form, of one out of what seem several simultaneously possible objects or trains of thought. Focalization, concentration, of consciousness are of its essence. It implies withdrawal from some things in order to deal effectively with others."[5]

Problems are bound to arise when attempting to measure a loosely defined concept such as attention or differentiating between attention and perception.[6, 7] However, the fundamental fact regarding our understanding of attention is that of *selection*. The mind is not fully aware of all things at once, but somehow focuses on one thing at a time.[8, 9] If the musician thinks about his health or tax problems when playing, he is likely to hit a wrong note.[10]

Normally, social conventions and neurobiological-orienting mechanisms cause people to immediately turn their attention to an individual who comes into their presence and addresses them. Both interruptions (an immediate cognitive need) and distractions (an ongoing cognitive need) can cause us to lose our place in a current task and overlook a required action.[3] The use of a checklist and the sterile cockpit can help keep attention focused on completing the steps of the task at hand.

---

from a previous mastectomy? Have nurses ever forgotten to remove sharps from the patient's bed or bedside? Have nurses ever inserted a smaller gauged catheter only to discover that the patient will be receiving blood transfusions? If you can answer no to all of the above, then I agree, there is no need for the checklist. If, on the other hand, you acknowledge the existence of such events, then read on.

Figure 9.2 is an example of an IV insertion checklist. Notice the format: clear, concise, and easy to read. Here is how it would be used in practice. The nurse gathers appropriate supplies, enters the patient's room and uses two identifiers to be sure she has the right patient. She checks the order, briefs the patient on what she is about to do, and verifies that needle sticks and venipunctures are not contraindicated on either arm. **Then, before actually inserting the catheter**, she references the "Before Insertion" part of the read and verify checklist; this takes about five to seven seconds to do. After the catheter is inserted the nurse then secures, dresses and labels the IV site, programs the infusion pump, documents the start date, and disposes of sharps and trash. **Then, before leaving the patient's room**, she references the "After Insertion" part of the read and verify checklist. Most times, all the steps are completed correctly, but perhaps the nurse may discover that she has left out an important step, the result of a cognitive lapse, fatigue, or an environmental distraction. ◆

FIGURE
9.2

IV Insertion Checklist

Before Insertion

Patient Identification...CONFIRMED
Correct Side ....CONFIRMED
Catheter Size..CONFIRMED
Equipment...AT BEDSIDE
IV Fluids..CONFIRMED
Patient ....BRIEFED

After Insertion

Tourniquet...REMOVED
Line ....FLUSHED
Pump..SET (with fluids)
Sharps ....DISPOSED
Site ....LABELED
Documentation..COMPLETE

Notice one other very important feature about the format of this checklist. Rather than put directives in a sentence that must be read by the user, it simply provides a **noun on the left with dots that lead you to an action on the right**. This is most consistent with the airline style that I believe creates optimal utility. For example rather than say "Obtain equipment at the bedside" or "Remove the tourniquet from patient," only the word "Equipment" and "Tourniquet" appears on the left with the corresponding action far to the right. This format is especially useful if

◆ Sidebar 9.3
A task deferred is a task denied

A common form of human attention deficient related error has occurred when a task is interrupted and one forgets to resume the deferred task.[11] A typical manifestation is that as individuals find themselves overwhelmed by increases in workload (i.e., the number of concurrent task demands), they seek to reduce cognitive demands by abandoning a strategic management of their situation and simply react to each new task demand as it is presented.[12] Keeping track of the status of each of the individual tasks on hold itself becomes a metatask. Remembering to remember (prospective memory) then competes with the original task(s) for the limited cognitive resources of working memory and attention. Thus, deferring a task after being interrupted creates a considerable risk that the original task(s) will be entirely forgotten. Even interrupting a habitual and familiar task such as veinipuncture for an appreciable period increases the risk of forgetting to return to the interrupted task to complete an essential step, especially when attention is drawn to one demanding task after another.[3]

the checklist is used in a **challenge – response** manner by more than one individual. With the challenge – response method, one clinician will read the noun on the left aloud, and another clinician will respond with the action on the right.

Obviously not all nursing tasks require a checklist; in fact, we can cause great difficulty for ourselves as clinicians by developing too many of them. However, as nurses continue to operate in a complex and fast-paced environment, the chance for omissions with routine procedural events is ever present. For patients, the stakes are high, because small omissions place them at risk, and often become bigger problems. The appropriate use of a well-constructed read and verify checklist, thoughtfully applied to **select** routine tasks can reduce these risks.

Read and do checklists

Read and do checklists are used in situations that are more critical such as rapidly changing scenarios, critical events, abnormalities, and emergencies. Unlike routine scenarios, in emergent situations, individuals can experience strong physiologic reactions such as fear or anxiety that must be managed while still performing required tasks. The stress of an emergency can make it extremely difficult to recall items from memory; the ability to assess and critically think can be negatively affected which reduces situational awareness as the scenario unfolds. Critical situations and emergencies often present a complex set of variables and the appropriate response may depend on the presence or absence of specific circumstances. Accurate analysis is required to select the most appropriate course of action. Read and do checklists allow humans to move through this process by providing guidance and direction so that assessments and analysis are focused on the right things, and the actions taken are suitable for the conditions experienced. With read and do checklists, beyond a few initial procedural items that **"may"** be carried out from memory, all items are read directly from the checklist, then carried out, one by one. All that is required is to follow the checklist until completion. This is an important distinction from the read and verify checklist in terms of both use and construction.

In the cockpit, a situation that calls for the use of a read and do checklist may be an engine failure or malfunction of a specific component or system on the airplane. Once the malfunction or failure is identified, a book with multiple read and do checklists for each situation is referenced, the appropriate one found and then followed by the crew. On the nursing unit, there are many critical scenarios that will benefit from the appropriate use of a well constructed read and do checklist. Before we get to that, let's first look at the construction and presentation of such a checklist.

In the following section, two examples of read and do checklists are presented. Once again, disregard the aviation content and focus in on the way the checklist is presented. Figure 9.3 depicts a generic engine fire checklist. Notice now that there *is* verbiage and instruction which present decision points for the user based on the presence or absence of certain conditions. Observe that the right side of the checklist for the most part is telling the user to

FIGURE
9.3

Engine Fire Checklist

Engine Fire Checklist

Essential Power Selector..OPERATING GEN

Thrust Lever ....CLOSE

Start Lever.. CUTOFF

Engine Fire Switch..PULL

- *If fire warning light remains illuminated*

Bottle Discharge Switch...PUSH

Bottle Discharge Light... CHECK ON

Bottle Transfer Switch...TRANSFER

- *If after 30 seconds the fire warning light remains illuminated*

Bottle Discharge Switch ....PUSH

Bottle Discharge Light.. CHECK ON

- *If fire warning light extinguished, proceed to One Engine Inoperative Checklist on Page E-6*

- *If fire warning remains illuminated PROCEED TO NEAREST SUITABLE AIRPORT AND LAND AS SOON AS POSSIBLE. Continue below...*

Galley Power Switch.. SELECT OFF

Cargo Heat Outflow Switch (If Applicable)...CLOSE

Pack Switch .... SELECT OFF

Generator Field...CHECK TRIPPED

Electrical Load..CHECK AND MONITOR

Fuel Shutoff Switch..CLOSE

Hydraulic System A Fluid Shutoff Switch ....CLOSE

Engine Bleed Air Switch..CLOSE

Wing & Engine Inlet Anti-Ice Switches (Affected Engine) .... SELECT OFF

- *Proceed to One Engine Inoperative / Landing Checklist on Page E-7*

do something, to "check," "pull," or "close" an item in real time. Nothing is presented in the past tense and the feel of the checklist is that the user is following a set of instructions, which, of course, is the intent. Engine failure and other emergencies are not "routine"; they are low frequency–high risk events, much like a code blue on a general med–surg unit. No one should expect the user to resolve these situations completely from memory.

Earlier I mentioned that with read and do checklists, there are a few procedural items that **"may"** be carried out from memory. These items are presented in bold face in Figure 9.3. Some airlines require that pilots memorize these bold faced items; others strongly discourage any memorization in such circumstances. The idea behind memorizing bold faced items is that there are a few time critical tasks that should be accomplished without delay. The wisdom in discouraging memorization is that when the rare emergency happens, the shock factor, the physiologic reactions that must be quelled, greatly hinder recall anyway so it's best to take a take a deep breath and go to the checklist. My personal opinion, based largely from experiencing and watching flight crews perform during multiple emergencies in a simulator, is that there are a few procedural actions that people can recall; beyond that all bets are off. For example, if a pilot experiences the failure of an engine on takeoff, he/she will press the appropriate rudder pedal with the foot to maintain control of the aircraft. This is something that is accomplished almost naturally as a matter of procedure, the result of repetition and training. After this the pilot can reference a checklist to know exactly what to do next and in what sequence. This would be analogous to a med–surg nurse starting CPR and calling a code when discovering a lifeless patient. Even though there may be difficulty recalling exactly what to do next and in what sequence, starting CPR and calling for the Code Team is something that can be easily remembered, also the result of training and repetition. In the end, there is no absolute when it comes to recall, therefore read and do checklists should present **all** information in an easy to follow step by step fashion, so the user can accomplish **all** tasks without relying on memory.

Figure 9.4 depicts another format for the read and do checklist often used in aviation. Notice the expanded verbiage and decision tree format. When presented this way, it is clear that memorizing the steps and decision points in a practical sense is not a real option.

FIGURE
9.4

Engine Fire Checklist: Read and Do

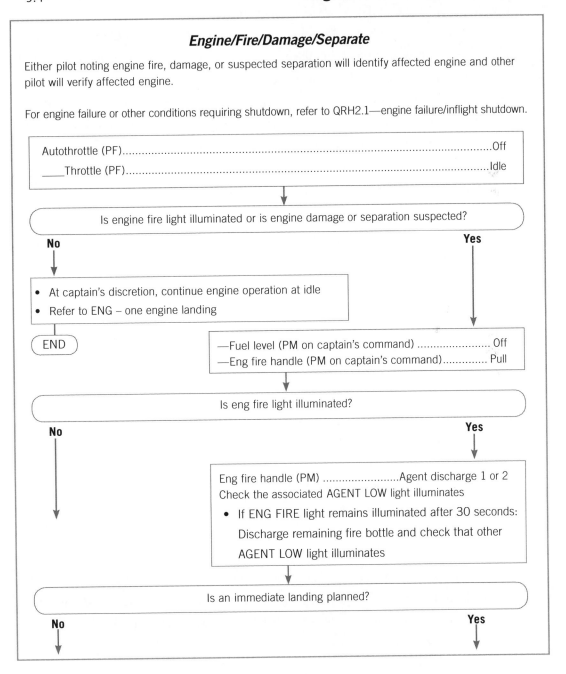

Engine/Fire/Damage/Separate

Either pilot noting engine fire, damage, or suspected separation will identify affected engine and other pilot will verify affected engine.

For engine failure or other conditions requiring shutdown, refer to QRH2.1—engine failure/inflight shutdown.

Autothrottle (PF)..Off
____Throttle (PF)..Idle

Is engine fire light illuminated or is engine damage or separation suspected?

No   **Yes**

- At captain's discretion, continue engine operation at idle
- Refer to ENG – one engine landing

END

—Fuel level (PM on captain's command) .... Off
—Eng fire handle (PM on captain's command)............. Pull

Is eng fire light illuminated?

No   **Yes**

Eng fire handle (PM) ....Agent discharge 1 or 2
Check the associated AGENT LOW light illuminates
- If ENG FIRE light remains illuminated after 30 seconds: Discharge remaining fire bottle and check that other AGENT LOW light illuminates

Is an immediate landing planned?

No   **Yes**

Read and Do Checklists in Nursing

A good example of read and do checklists in nursing are the advanced cardiac life support (ACLS) algorithms found in the *American Heart Association Handbook of Emergency Cardio-vascular Care for Healthcare Providers*. The book uses reference tabs so that particular critical situations requiring action can be easily found. This feels very natural to me because it is very much like the indexed book of read and do checklists one finds in the cockpit of an airliner. Although they are termed algorithms, not checklists, the feel and presentation resembles the read and do checklists presented in this chapter; and, while the format could be improved for the sake of usability (nouns on the left and actions on the right), these are excellent tools to support human memory in specific critical cardiovascular events.

The typical multibed medical surgical unit is often a place where one can find a mix of staff in terms of licensure and experience. For those med–surg veterans out there, you know that it is common to have patients residing on your unit who are acutely ill, often requiring intense monitoring on the bubble between the general ward and a step down or intensive care unit. You know what it's like when you walk into a room and find the patient in a state of general decline: unstable vital signs, changes in mental status, labored breathing, and pallor. Often the patient does not have cardiac monitoring, so you can't be immediately sure what's happening. Over the years, you have learned from experience what to do, how to respond, what to look for, but even so there are still times where situations can become confusing and even chaotic. If you are a neophyte nurse within your first year of practice, a situation like this can be extremely difficult to discern and manage. The patient's outcome should not be solely dependent on the experience level of the nurse that happens to be taking care of him or her at a given moment. The clinical response should be consistent, regardless of personnel. A read and do checklist applied to this situation can go a long way toward reaching that consistency. I envision an **"Unstable Patient" Checklist** to guide nursing assessments and actions in this critical scenario. Figure 9.5 presents a general example that can be modified to fit specific patient populations and organizational policies. Notice in this example the existence of other read and do checklists that are referenced within.

FIGURE
9.5

Unstable Patient Checklist

Unstable Patient (Unmonitored)

Not Responsive, Not Breathing and Pulseless

Code Blue...**ACTIVATE**

CPR ....**INITIATE**

- Assign staff member to complete "FIRST RESPONDER CHECKLIST" page 2

SOB or Respiratory Difficulty

HOB ....REPOSITION

Airway...MAINTAIN AND CHECK FOR OBSTRUCTION

Airway...SUCTION AS NECESSARY

O_2 Sat...CHECK

Oxygen...APPLY IF **O_2 SAT < 90%**

- If O_2 sat > 90%, still apply Oxygen as needed

- If COPD Patient do not apply 100% Oxygen

Resp Rate ....CHECK

Oxygen... APPLY IF **< 8/min or > 28/min**

- If < 8/minute and not arousable, consider Ambu Bag

Rapid Response Team ....CONSIDER

Physician ....NOTIFY

Perfusion Difficulty

Bedside Heart Monitor...OBTAIN AND MONITOR

Heart Rate .... CHECK IF **< 50/min or > 120/min**

- If < 50 assess LOC

- If > 120 assess level and location of pain

- If Chest Pain refer to "CHEST PAIN CHECKLIST" page 6

FIGURE
9.5

Unstable Patient Checklist (cont.)

Blood Pressure.. CHECK IF **< 90 mmHg or > 180 mmHg**

Urine Output .... CHECK IF **< 50cc / 4 hours**

IV Access.. ESTABLISH

Oxygen... APPLY AS NECESSARY

Rapid Response Team ....CONSIDER

Physician .... NOTIFY

Difficult to Arouse

Verbal or Tactile Stimulus.. ATTEMPT

Airway.. MAINTAIN

Vital Signs .... CHECK

Oxygen...APPLY IF **O$_2$ SAT < 90**

- *If sat > 90, still apply Oxygen if needed*

- *If COPD patient do not apply 100% O$_2$*

IV Access..ESTABLISH

Bedside Heart Monitor..OBTAIN AND MONITOR

Recent Narcotics...VERIFY AND CONSIDER NARCAN

Diabetic Patient.. VERIFY AND CONSIDER HYPOGLYCEMIA

- Check Blood Glucose. If < 60 go to "HYPOGLYCEMIA CHECKLIST" Page 9

Rapid Response Team ....CONSIDER

Physician .... NOTIFY

End of Checklist

Source: Adapted from material from the Institute for Healthcare Improvement, the Agency for Healthcare Research, and suggestions from Dr. Douglas E. Paull, MD

In the situation previously discussed, where a nurse discovers a lifeless patient and promptly snaps into action by calling a code and starting CPR, these two actions are almost naturally recalled. But what happens next? On an inpatient unit, several minutes can elapse before the hospital ACLS team arrives. What happens within that window of time, and whether specific actions are completed in an organized and timely fashion, can be the difference between a trip to the ICU or a trip to the morgue for the patient. This is a perfect situation for a **read and do "First Responder Checklist"** for nurses practicing in the medical–surgical specialty as these units commonly utilize staff not certified in ACLS protocol. The checklist guides the first responders on appropriate actions so that when the ACLS team arrives, all elements are in place for the timely administration of drugs, early defibrillation, and airway support, thus giving the patient a better chance for survival. For example, elements like IV access, endotracheal intubation supplies, suction set up, oxygen, defibrillator, heart monitor leads, and emergency drugs can be referenced on the checklist then readied and/or implemented within a few minutes while CPR is first being delivered.

There are many other opportunities to develop both read and verify and read and do checklists to support decision making and situational awareness in nursing practice. Optimally, I would love to see all nurses carrying with them a standardized pocket manual divided into two sections. The first section would be termed "Routine Procedures" and have within it specific read and verify checklists. The second section would be termed "Emergency/Critical Event Procedures" and comprised of relevant read and do checklists. The checklist manual could be tailored to particular units depending on patient population. Pilots always have such a manual at their disposal when in the cockpit to ensure procedural accuracy and flight safety; it makes sense for nurses to follow suit in the interest of patient safety.

When the philosophy does not match the task

The checklist philosophy used for development must match the task; if not, then clinicians will reject them because they're too difficult to use. As I mentioned in Chapter 8, Theresa Pape is a visionary as she applied the sterile cockpit concept directly to medication administration on the med–surg unit. One of the elements in her study was the use of a medication delivery checklist. Based on her results and discussion, the checklist was not widely used or accepted. Why was this case? Let's look at her checklist in Figure 9.6.

FIGURE
9.6

Medication Administration Checklist

Medication administration checklist for focused protocol	Medication administration checklist for med-safe focused protocol with vest

1. Verify all assigned patients MAR forms with MD orders.
2. DO NOT engage in conversation not pertaining to medication delivery.
3. DO NOT allow interruptions of distractions while administering medication.
  a. Hold your hand up and verbalize the need for no interruptions or distractions
  b. Other staff members "field" phones calls and interruptions for nurse.
4. Prioritize tasks.
5. Obtain medication and verify with MAR.
6. Look at items being read.
7. Use 7 rights: Right drug, right patient, right dose, right time, right route, right reason, right documentation.
8. Administer medications to only one patient at a time.
  a. Right patient
9. Take MAR and unit-dose packets to bedside.
  a. Verify patient's armband name and MD name with exact spelling on MAR.
  b. Ask patient to state name.
10. Read medication name aloud to patient while opening unit-dose packet.
11. Correctly document medications given.
12. Continue with second patient, etc.
	1. Verify all assigned patients MAR forms with MD orders.
	2. Place Medsafe vest on self.
	3. DO NOT engage in conversation not pertaining to medication delivery.
	4. DO NOT allow interruptions of distractions while administering medication.
	  a. State, "Medsafe protocol is being followed at present."
	  b. Other staff members "field" phones calls and interruptions for Medsafe nurse.
	5. Prioritize tasks.
	6. Obtain medication and verify with MAR.
	7. Look at items being read.
	8. Use 7 rights: Right drug, right patient, right dose, right time, right route, right reason, right documentation.
	9. Administer medications to only one patient at a time.
	  a. Right patient
	10. Take MAR and unit-dose packets to bedside.
	  a. Verify patient's armband name and MD name with exact spelling on MAR.
	  b. Ask patient to state name.
	11. Read medication name aloud to patient while opening unit-dose packet.
	12. Correctly document medications given.
	13. Continue with second patient, etc.

Source: Pape, T.M. 2003. Applying airline safety practices to medication administration. Reprinted from MEDSURG Nursing, 2003, Volume 12, Number 2, p. 77–93. Reprinted with permission of the publisher, Jannetti Publications, Inc., Pitman, NJ.

One reason might be that the checklist is laden with instructions that really don't need to be there. For example: "Prioritize tasks," "Look at items being read," "Place vest on self," and "Do not engage in conversation not pertaining to medication delivery." These are all actions that are self-evident and will be accomplished automatically, by the medication nurse; placing them on the checklist clutters things up and adds a burden to the user. The need to spell things out in such a detailed fashion can be saved for policy and procedure manuals, which are the basis for the checklist.

Perhaps the most relevant problem with this well-intentioned checklist is that there is an obvious mismatch between the work it was intended for and the philosophy used to develop it. Medication administration is a routine task; frequently accomplished routine tasks match well with checklists designed for a read and verify methodology. This checklist is presented in a read and do fashion with multiple numbered lines of instructions, some with secondary instructions beneath. As we discussed, read and do checklists are best used in emergency situations where the user reads and does one line at a time. Chances are, nurses administering medications with this type of checklist would find it to be cumbersome, perhaps adding to their mental load. This is not a criticism of Pape's work; on the contrary, the fact that she was using a checklist at all is something to celebrate.

In Figure 9.7, I offer a rework of Theresa Pape's medication administration checklist.

FIGURE
9.7

Medication Administration Checklist

Medication Administration MedSafe – Focused Protocol

Before Administration:

Medication Orders ....VERIFIED IN LAST 24 HRS BY RN
Medsafe Vest .... ON

During Administration:

MAR ....AT BEDSIDE
Patient Identified X 2 .... COMPLETE
Allergies.. VERIFIED
Medication .... CHECKED WITH MAR
Dose .... CHECKED
Route.. CHECKED
Time Due.. WITHIN LIMITS
Indicated for this Patient.. CHECKED

After Administration:

Documentation... COMPLETE

Moving Forward

In 2009, the World Health Organization published a global study that demonstrated statistically significant reductions in postoperative complications and mortality with the use of a surgical safety checklist. The checklist was used prior to anesthesia induction, prior to incision, and prior to transfer out of the operating room for postanesthesia recovery. In the same year, Dr. Atul Gawande published his book *The Checklist Manifesto: How to Get Things Right.*

The attention and focus on using checklists to keep patients safe will continue to build, as it should. Nurses will be encouraged, perhaps required, to expand checklist implementation in practice. It is therefore paramount that nursing staff at the front line be intimately involved in checklist development, matching checklist structure and presentation to the targeted clinical task. This will ensure that standardization, situational awareness, and human memory will be supported, not hindered, and that checklists will fit the unique environment in which nurses practice.

References

1.   Sine, D., and G. Sculli. Just Checking: Using Team Briefings to Improve Patient Safety. *Healthbeat, 2010. 9*(3): p. 4–6.

2.   Norman, D.A., *The Design of Everyday Things*. 1990, New York: Doubleday.

3.   Loukopoulos, L., R. Dismukes, and I. Barshi, *The Multitaskng Myth*. 2009, Burlington, VT: Ashgate.

4.   Winters, D.D., A.P. Gurses, H. Lehmann, et al. Clinical review: Checklists - translating evidence into practice. *Critical Care, 2009. 13*(6): p. 210.

5.   James, W., *The Principles of Psychology*. (1890) 1999, New York Henry Holt.

6.   Saunders, A.F., *Elements of Human Performance: Reaction Processes and Attention in Human Skill.* 1998, Mahwah, NJ: Lawrence Erlbaum Associates.

7.   Dallenbach, K.M., *Attributive vs. cognitive clearness. Journal of Experimental Psychology, 3*(3): p. 183–230.

8.   Bacon, W.F. *What Everyone Knows about Attention*. 1995 [cited AAAI Technical Report SS-95-05]; Available from: *www.aaai.org/Papers/Symposia/Spring/1995/SS-95-05/SS95-05-001.pdf.*

9.   Csikszentmihalyi, M., *Flow: The Psychology of Optimal Experience*. 1990, New York: Harper.

10.   Csikszentmihalyi, M., *Creativity: Flow and the Psychology of Discovery and Invention*. 1996, New York: HarperCollins.

11.   Reason, J., Combating omission errors through task analysis and good reminders. *Quality and Safety in Health Care, 2002. 11*: p. 40–44.

12.   Dismukes, R., B. Berman, and L. Loukopoulous, *The Limits of Expertise: Rethinking Pilot Error and the Causes of Airlines Accidents*. 2007, Aldershot, United Kingdom: Ashgate.

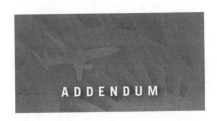

Building an Airline-Based Recurrent Training Model for Nursing Practice

Vigilance: A state of being alert, watchful, attentive, and wary of potential dangers
Complacency: A feeling of quiet pleasure or security, often while unaware of some potential danger

Take a look at Figure A.1, which depicts a complacency-vigilance continuum. Vigilance is essential for safety. When professionals undergo initial training and validation, they reside on the left side of the continuum where vigilance is the highest. As time passes, the natural human tendency is to migrate to the right of the continuum, becoming less vigilant. Over longer periods of time, professionals become comfortable, moving into complacency. Some force or event is required to move the professional back to the vigilance side of the continuum from which point the migration begins again. **Professional life, therefore, is constant movement from complacency to vigilance and back again.**

Take the case of a new nurse, Jim, just starting in a staff position on a medical–surgical unit. Jim has just completed rigorous training and standardized board exams. He is current and versed in the latest editions of pharmacologic and medical–surgical texts and regularly reads professional nursing journals. While working on the unit, Jim places great effort in avoiding error. He will check and double-check with available resources (pharmacy, nurse colleagues, etc.) before making decisions. He ensures he is well rested when practicing, avoiding alcohol and late nights on the town before duty periods. This nurse is truly vigilant.

At the six-month point, things change somewhat. Jim is getting the hang of things and is much more comfortable managing the routine challenges of the work environment. Textbooks collect dust on the book shelf and the knowledge they contain begins to get hazy

Soaring to Success

FIGURE
A.1

Complacency Vigilance Continuum

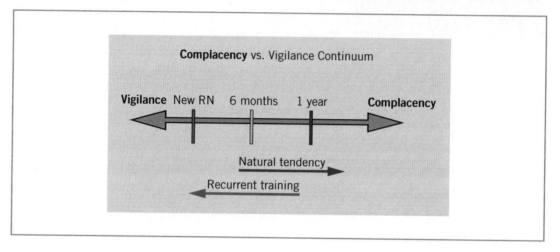

in his mind. Professional journals are read less often, and sleep may be sacrificed for a night out with friends. The nurse moves to the right on the continuum.

At the one-year point, Jim feels completely comfortable in his position. He carries out clinical policies while practicing but has difficulty recalling the reasons and theory behind such policies. Life on the unit becomes routine, he may no longer feel challenged, and defenses are relaxed. He is now complacent, residing on the right side of the continuum.

What will move Jim back to the vigilance side of the continuum? In nursing there is no mandated mechanism to do so and migration back to vigilance occurs randomly. Perhaps a medication error is made; maybe he is faced with an emergent situation and responds sluggishly, uncomfortably struggling to recall the appropriate steps to manage the situation. Possibly he witnesses someone else make a catastrophic error. These experiences have the same effect. They move him back to the left side of the continuum, back to vigilance. He emerges from the experience with a renewed sense of professionalism. The journals and textbooks are once again opened, policies are reviewed, and actions that have become routine are again connected with the theory and knowledge that supports them.

Unfortunately, the dominant mechanism to drive professional nurses back to vigilance is haphazard and random, most often not the result of formal training, but of real-life clinical experiences. From the patient's perspective, this appears to be a somewhat risky proposition. It will better serve both patient and nurse to develop a formal recurrent training and performance checking modality such as those that exist at the airlines. The premise is that **as professionals feel the pressure associated with an upcoming training and performance evaluation event, pertinent policies, procedures and standards are thoroughly reviewed.**

Training Module

Airlines use recurrent (refresher) training and performance checking to counter the natural human tendency toward complacency and ensure pilot proficiency. The training model is called the Airline Qualification Program (AQP). AQP guidelines have replaced older Federal Aviation Administration (FAA) regulations and provide airlines with complete flexibility and autonomy in determining how training will be structured, and what the most appropriate intervals between recurrent training events should be. The AQP program is a movement toward best practices (something we discuss a lot in nursing) in the maintenance of a pilot's professional competence. For example airlines use the results of actual pilot performance evaluations to determine the optimal amount of time that should elapse between recurrent training events.

Figure A.2 is a general example of an AQP template found at U.S. airlines. This is based on a 12-month training cycle. This template provides an excellent basis for a similar training program in professional nursing. Key points on the airline training timeline are presented along with proposed nursing equivalents. Figure A.3 provides complete descriptions of both the AQP terms and nursing equivalents. **A precondition for all nursing equivalent training is that nurses will not participate in any training event unless they are completely free**

Soaring to Success

from the responsibilities of patient care. As is the case with the airlines, training events are considered duty time.

FIGURE
A.2

Airline vs. Nursing Qualification Program

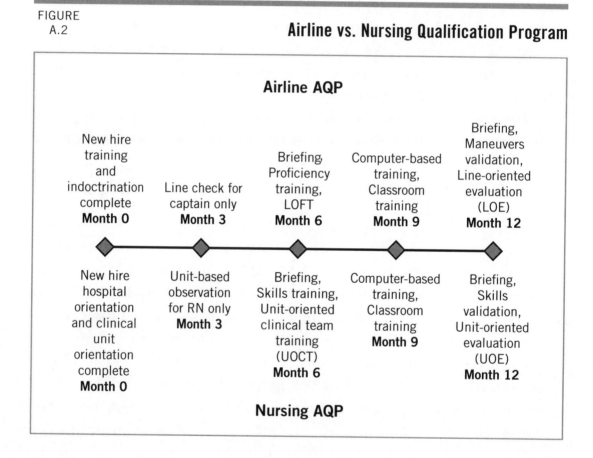

The nursing AQP Equivalent is a proposed guideline that is a departure from business as usual. Its use will require not only additional resources, but a significant commitment on the part of healthcare and nursing leadership. High-reliability cultures continuously train personnel using CRM and simulation.[1] If we are to truly achieve "high reliability" in patient care, we would be wise to create a culture that embraces perpetual training, practice, briefing and competency evaluation.

Nursing AQP Equivalent

Airline AQP	Nursing AQP Equivalent
Proficiency training: Pilots practice normal maneuvers, as well as the management of the aircraft during system malfunctions and failures in a full-motion aircraft simulator. It is practice only, and no formal evaluation takes place.	**Skills proficiency training:** Nurses practice technical and patient assessment skills specific to their patient population. Training occurs using a patient simulator or other simulation devices specific to the skill be practiced (e.g., intravenous arm). Nurses also practice using equipment necessary for the care of patients on the unit, such as hospital beds, IV pumps, glucose monitoring meters, chest tubes, nebulizers, etc. It is practice, and no formal evaluation takes place.
Line-oriented flight training (LOFT): Rather than practice specific maneuvers, pilots work together as a crew and fly a normal flight just like they would in the real world (represented by the word "line"). They experience a malfunction and have to use technical knowledge and CRM to manage the situation safely. This takes place in a static or full motion flight simulator. It important to clarify that in LOFT, pilots will not be given unrealistic or multiple malfunctions that in all probability will never occur in day-to-day operations. The purpose of LOFT is to train in normal "line" operations. It is practice, and no formal evaluation takes place.	**Unit-oriented clinical team training (UOCT):** Nurses train with a multidisciplinary team of unit personnel (RN, LPN, physicians, and nursing assistants) using a patient simulator. The clinical scenario reflects a common clinical problem specific to the unit. Unrealistic or unusual clinical scenarios are not given in the UOCT. The purpose is for the team to manage a patient problems found in day-to-day operations using technical knowledge and CRM. It is practice, and no formal evaluation takes place.
Maneuvers validation: Pilots perform and are validated on normal maneuvers as well as the management of the aircraft during system malfunctions and failures. This is an assessment, not practice. If a pilot has trouble completing a specific maneuver, then he or she can be retrained on the spot and attempt validation again. If the pilot does not complete validation, more extensive retraining is required.	**Skills validation:** Nurses perform and are validated on technical and patient assessment skills specific to their patient population. The validation takes place using a patient simulator or other simulation devices specific to the skill be practiced (e.g., intravenous arm). Nurses also are validated on the use of equipment necessary for the care of patients on the unit such as hospital beds, IV pumps, glucose monitoring meters, chest tubes, nebulizers, etc. This is a proficiency assessment, not practice. If a nurse has trouble with a specific assessment or technical skill, retraining takes place until comfortable proficiency is attained.

Soaring to Success

Nursing AQP Equivalent *(cont.)*

Airline AQP	Nursing AQP Equivalent
Line-oriented evaluation (LOE): Pilots are evaluated individually and as a crew on a LOFT type scenario. This is performance checking, not practice. No retraining occurs during an LOE. If a pilot is unsatisfactory on any component of the LOE, the event is unsatisfactory and more extensive retraining is required. The LOE is the "check ride" discussed in Chapter 1.	**Unit-oriented evaluations (UOE):** Nurses are evaluated individually and as a member of a multidisciplinary team in the management on a UOCT type scenario. Individual skills in clinical knowledge, patient assessment, and CRM are evaluated. This is performance checking, not practice. If a nurse is unsatisfactory on any component of the UOE, the event is unsatisfactory and more extensive supportive retraining is required.
Classroom training: Pilots sit in a classroom setting to review airlines policies and procedures. Usually a full day.	**Classroom training:** Nurses are free from the responsibilities of patient care and receive training in a comfortable professional learning environment. Patient care and regulatory compliance policies are reviewed. Usually a full day.
Computer-based training: Pilots complete computer-based self-study and testing on aircraft systems and general airline policies and procedures.	**Computer-based training:** Nurses complete computer-based self-study and testing on recurring compliance requirements. Computer modules on pathophysiology, disease management, and pharmacology are also included.
Briefings: Conducted by the instructor with the crew. This occurs in conjunction with a simulation event (training, validation, or evaluation). Often covers important safety topics or changes and updates to operating procedures. Also reviews content that will be covered in the upcoming simulation session.	**Briefings:** Conducted by the nurse educator with individual nurses or multidisciplinary team prior to patient simulation events (training, validation or evaluation). Often covers important safety topics or changes and updates to policies and procedures. Also reviews content that will be covered in the upcoming simulation session.
Debriefing: Occurs postsimulation session to review performance.	**Debriefing:** Occurs postsimulation session to review performance.
Line check: The captain of the aircraft is observed on the line in the aircraft in revenue operations. This is a performance checking event. If the line check is not satisfactory, the pilot is taken off line and is retrained.	**Unit-based observation:** RNs are observed for a specified time period (minimum one hour) conducting patient care on the unit. The observation period begins from the time the nurse receives change of shift report and includes specified performance elements such as initial patient assessment and medication administration. This is a performance checking event. If the unit-based observation is not satisfactory, the nurse is given supportive retraining.

Soaring to Success

Reference

1. Gaba, D.M. 2004. The future vision of simulation in healthcare. *Qual. Saf. Health Care, 13,* i2–i10.

2. Conversation with Edwin L. Garbutt, ATP.

3. Conversation with Randy Hamilton, ATP.

FREE HEALTHCARE COMPLIANCE AND MANAGEMENT RESOURCES!

Need to control expenses yet stay current with critical issues?

Get timely help with FREE e-mail newsletters from HCPro, Inc., the leader in healthcare compliance education. Offering numerous free electronic publications covering a wide variety of essential topics, you'll find just the right e-newsletter to help you stay current, informed, and effective. All you have to do is sign up!

With your FREE subscriptions, you'll also receive the following:

- Timely information, to be read when convenient with your schedule
- Expert analysis you can count on
- Focused and relevant commentary
- Tips to make your daily tasks easier

And here's the best part: There's no further obligation—just a complimentary resource to help you get through your daily challenges.

It's easy. Visit *www.hcmarketplace.com/free/e-newsletters* to register for as many free e-newsletters as you'd like, and let us do the rest.

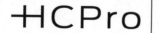

HCPro | Insight for healthcare compliance and management